Joseph
May 11, 1993
Las Vegas

Y0-ASQ-320

Remembrances in *Endocrinology*

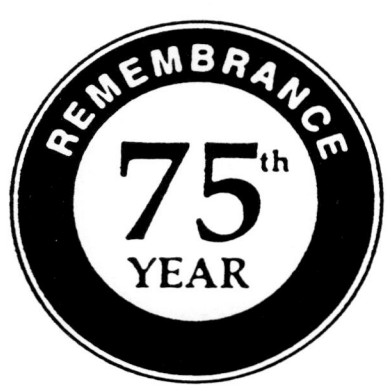

An Endocrine Society History of the Study of Endocrinology and its Practitioners

© Copyright 1993 The Endocrine Society.

All rights reserved. The reproduction or utilization of this work in any form or in any electronic, mechanical, or other means, now known or hereafter invented, including photocopying or recording and in any information storage or retrieval system is forbidden except as may be expressly permitted by the 1976 Copyright Act or by permission of the publisher.

ISBN 1-879225-09-3

Published by The Endocrine Society Press, 9650 Rockville Pike, Bethesda, MD 20814

Grateful acknowledgement is made to the contributors of the chapters herein, to P. Michael Conn, Ph.D., former Editor-in-Chief of *Endocrinology*, and to Maggie Haworth.

Printed in the United States on acid free paper.

Remembrances in *Endocrinology*: An Endocrine Society History of the Study of Endocrinology and its Practitioners

Introduction	P. Michael Conn	1

1991

Letter to the Readers (Vol. 129, No. 1)	P. Michael Conn	2
Endocrinology: Some Growing Pains (Vol. 129, No. 1)	Roy O. Greep	3
Growth of The Endocrine Society Journals (Vol. 129, No. 1)	Delbert A. Fisher	5
From Enzyme to Transport and back to Enzyme – Insulin Action over Forty Years (Vol. 129, No. 1)	Joseph Larner	8
Remembrances of the Meadowbrook Conferences – When Steroids Came to DNA (Vol. 129, No. 2)	Arun K. Roy	11
Remembrances of Contributions of Philip Smith and Bernardo Houssay to the Development of Neuroendocrinology (Vol. 129, No. 2)	Charles H. Sawyer	13
Glycoprotein Hormones Were Always Composed of Subunits – We Just Had to Find Out the Hard Way (Vol. 129, No. 2)	Harold Papkoff	15
Origin of the Hormone Action Gordon Research Conference (Vol. 129, No. 3)	James R. Florini	18
History of the Gordon Conference on Hormone Action (Vol. 129, No. 3)	Frances Finn	22
Memoir – The Beginning of Oral Contraceptives (Vol. 129, No. 3)	Richard A. Edgren	25
The 1959 West Point Conference on Mechanisms Concerned with Conception: A Landmark Event in Endocrinology (Vol. 129, No. 3)	William Hansel	27
The Backstage Story of the Discovery of LHRH (Vol. 129, No. 4)	Akira Arimura	28
Why I was Told not to Study Inhibin and What I did about it (Vol. 129, No. 4)	Neena B. Schwartz	31
Remembrance of H.W. Magoun's Contributions to the Development of Neuroendocrinology (Vol. 129, No. 4)	Charles H. Sawyer	33
Remembrance Project: Origins of RIA (Vol. 129, No. 4)	Rosalyn S. Yalow	35
Henry Stanley Plummer (Vol. 129, No. 5)	William M. McConahey and Donald S. Pady	37
Remembrance of Dr. Alfred Jost (Vol. 129, No. 5)	Nathalie Josso	40
The Early Days of Steroid Radioimmunoassays at the Worcester Foundation (Vol. 129, No. 5)	Andrzej Bartke	43

The Beginnings of an Endocrinologist (Vol. 129, No. 6)	Martin Rodbell	45
Peptide and Protein Hormones – from Biological Definitions to Chemical Compounds (Vol. 129, No. 6)	John G. Pierce	47
A Footnote to Pituitary Transplantation Research (Vol. 129, No. 6)	John W. Everett	49
The Long and Evans Monograph on the Estrous Cycle in the Rat (Vol. 129, No. 6)	Leslie L. Bennett	50

1992

Remembrances of Our Founders: Will Growth Factors, Oncogenes, Cytokines, and Gastrointestinal Hormones Return Us to Our Beginnings? (Vol. 130, No. 1)	Judson J. Van Wyk	53
Alfred E. Mirsky and the Foundations of Molecular Biology and Neuroendocrinology (Vol. 130, No. 1)	Bruce S. McEwen and Caleb Finch	56
The Early History of the Releasing Factors (Vol. 130, No. 1)	Samuel M. McCann	58
Nettie Karpin Remembers... (Vol. 130, No. 2)	Nettie Karpin	60
A Failed Assay Opened a New Door in Growth Hormone Research (Vol. 130, No. 2)	William H. Daughaday	62
NIH Scientists Develop Specific Assays for Human Chorionic Gonadotropin (Vol. 130, No. 3)	Gary D. Hodgen	64
Reminiscences of the Twelfth Floor of the Clinical Center of NIH (circa 1965) (Vol. 130, No. 3)	Peter O. Kohler	67
Remembrance of an Unexpected Turn in the Road (Vol. 130, No. 4)	Jack H. Oppenheimer	69
Remembrance: Discovery of the Vitamin D Endocrine System (Vol. 130, No. 4)	Hector F. DeLuca	71
Remembrance: Steps Leading to the Identification, Purification, and Characterization of the Glucocorticoid Receptor (Vol. 130, No. 5)	Gerald Litwack	72
Remembrance: Scientific Contributions of Larry L. Ewing (1936–1990) (Vol. 130, No. 5)	Barry R. Zirkin	74
Remembrance: Neuroendocrinology and Aging. A Perspective (Vol. 130, No. 6)	Joseph Meites	77
Remembrance: Tracing the Glucose Tracer Dilution Technique for Measuring Glucose Turnover (Vol. 130, No. 6)	Norman Altszuler	79
Remembrance: Mort and Griff (Vol. 131, No. 1)	D. Lynn Loriaux	83

Remembrance: Leslie L. Iversen, Merck Sharp & Dohme Research Laboratories, Neuroscience Research Centre, Harlow, England. "The Axelrod Lab, 1964–1965" (Vol. 131, No. 1)	Leslie L. Iversen	86
The Concept of Negative Feedback – Moore and Price (Vol. 131, No. 2)	Darhl Foreman	87
Thyroxine Transport and the Free Hormone Hypothesis (Vol. 131, No. 2)	Jacob Robbins	90
Remembrance: Columbia University's Endocrine Journal Club (Vol. 131, No. 3)	Seymour Lieberman	92
Remembrance: The Discovery of the Hypothalamic Gonadotropin-Releasing Hormone Pulse Generator and of its Physiological Significance (Vol. 131, No. 3)	Ernst Knobil	94
Remembrance: Calcitonin: Discovery and Early Development (Vol. 131, No. 3)	D. Harold Copp	96
Remembrance: Gregory Pincus – Catalyst for Early Receptor Studies (Vol. 131, No. 4)	Elwood V. Jensen	98
Remembrance: The Introduction of Molecular Biology and Receptors into the Study of Hormone Action (Vol. 131, No. 4)	Jack Gorski	100
Remembrance: The Story of Inhibin – The Melbourne Version (Vol. 131, No. 4)	Henry Burger	102
Remembrance: Excerpta Memorabilia (Vol. 131, No. 4)	Robert L. Kroc	104
The Development of the Role of Hormones in Development – a Double Remembrance (Vol. 131, No. 5)	Howard A. Bern	105
Remembrance: Growing Up with the Pineal Gland: Early Recollections (Vol. 131, No. 5)	Russel J. Reiter	107
Remembrance: The Discovery of Growth Hormone (GH)-Releasing Hormone and GH Release-Inhibiting Hormone (Vol. 131, No. 5)	Samuel M. McCann	110
Remembrance for the Year 2016 (Vol. 131, No. 6)	P. Michael Conn	113

ADDITIONAL ACKNOWLEDGMENTS

Van Wyk
Figure 1: Excerpted from Endocrinology: The Glands and Their Functions by R.G. Hoskins, Copyright © 1941 by W.W. Norton & Company, Inc., Reprinted with permission of the publisher, W.W. Norton & Company, Inc.

Introduction

Beginning in July 1991 and continuing through December 1992, *Endocrinology* commemorated its 75th anniversary with the "Remembrance Project" in which we sought to create an informal history of our discipline as seen through the eyes of many individuals. Following are the Remembrances as they appeared in the individual issues during those eighteen months. Minor correction of fact and typography have been made. I hope you enjoy them.

P. Michael Conn

Letter to the Readers:

It is a great pleasure to be serving as Editor-in-Chief during the 75th anniversary of the Journal. Discussions of how best to celebrate this occasion began over 2 years ago. This Journal has, on two occasions, published histories of the Endocrine Society—one prepared by Hans Lisser (1) and one by Alfred Wilhelmi (2). These have emphasized the view that discrete events and specific people and occasions have existed which provide focal points and turning points in our profession. As a way of commemorating our anniversary we have sought to identify such events and individuals willing to share their remembrances of them with the readers of the Journal.

This "Remembrance Project" promises to provide insights into how we got where we are today. We have tried to provide a personal yet informal history, viewing the development of modern endocrinology and Endocrinology through the eyes of many people. We begin with three pieces—one by Dr. Roy Greep (a past editor of *Endocrinology*, viewing the trials of the Journal), one by Dr. Delbert Fisher (a past editor of *The Journal of Clinical Endocrinology and Metabolism*), and one by Dr. Joseph Larner (a leader in insulin action) dealing with how insulin mechanisms of action got here from there. I hope you enjoy these "Remembrances." Suggestions for others are, of course, welcome.

P. Michael Conn
Editor-in-Chief

References

1. Lisser H 1967 The Endocrine Society: the first forty years: 1917–1957. Endocrinology 80:5–28
2. Wilhelmi A 1988 The Endocrine Society: origin, organization, and institutions. Endocrinology 123:1–43

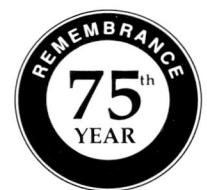

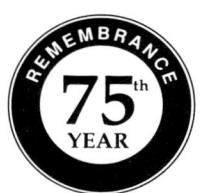

Endocrinology: Some Growing Pains*

Since *Endocrinology* is universally recognized as a prestigious and flourishing journal and shifts to a new Editor-in-Chief every fifth year, it would be a mistake to assume that these two circumstances have always existed. When I came aboard in 1952 at the invitation of Warren Nelson on behalf of the Society the fortunes of *Endocrinology* were at a low ebb. Gaps between the mailing of two or even three issues at one time ranged up to 6 months. The Publisher, C C Thomas, was threatening to pull out and many leading investigators were seeking other outlets for their important papers. As to term of service, Roy Hoskins, the first editor, served 25 yr, E. B. Astwood 2, Ed Dempsey 7, and myself 10. Whatever low points may be noted in the 75-yr history of this journal none can compare with its neonatal period when Hoskins had to pad the pages of what was then a quarterly with book reviews, abstracts from the world's literature, and Society news. His successor, Astwood, found the editorial demands on his time incompatible with those of stardom in thyroidology. Dempsey's situation developed coincident with his move to a new location with overwhelming administrative demands, coupled with a major shift in his field of interest, *i.e.* from endocrinology to electron microscopy. It was during my tenure with Al Albert at the helm of *The Journal of Endocrinology and Metabolism* (JCEM) and Rulon Rawson in charge of publications that the idea of changing editors every 5 yr was put into effect, thereby avoiding some of the perils of the past.

On my receipt of the files of *Endocrinology,* I found that they contained 89 unopened manuscripts and many more were languishing in the hands of the Editorial Board, whose distinguished and venerable members had no limitation on tenure of service. I originally planned to edit the journal out of my office at Harvard but the looming magnitude of effort made this an unlikely prospect. The services of a part-time secretary were critical but the Society's financial situation was abysmal. I did not mind volunteering my service but finding secretarial help on a charitable basis was to say the least unrewarding. In desperation I turned to a vulnerable source, my wife, Eunice. She agreed providing I do the dishes and so things went for a couple years.

Every evening I came home with a bulging briefcase, the contents of which required our attention until midnight or beyond. In those days all of the redactory work on galley and page proofs was done by me. Eunice did the typing, mailings, and record keeping. She also compiled the author index and I did the subject index. After a couple of years the Publication Committee, at Ted Astwood's insistence, put Eunice on a small salary. As a neighbor he knew the extent of her labors and the burning of midnight oil. This workload was relieved to some extent when in our final year (1962) publication of the Society's journals was taken over by J. B. Lippincott. In due course Eunice gained increasing but not lavish tangible support and even the editor came to rate a small annual lump sum. The psychological impact was greater that way than by receiving the same amount in driblets.

In an effort to enhance the quality of the journal I appointed a new Editorial Board of eager beavers, implored topnotch investigators to send me their best, and sought general cooperation in shortening the time of manuscript processing and publication time—a practice that persists to this day. I am pleased to note that our efforts began paying off for the Society almost immediately and continued to do so both financially and in terms of number of manuscripts submitted and number published each succeeding year. We had one big factor going in our favor, namely the arrival of significant federal support of biomedical research. Dare I recall that this bonanza of support was increasing at an average annual rate of 15% all during the fifties. This "Ask and thou shall be given" era couldn't last and didn't. It gave a tremendous boost to research, especially the basic variety. This trend can still be monitored by the heftiness of each new issue of *Endocrinology.*

Within the Society the pendulum of attention to clinical *vs.* fundamental interests has been swinging to and fro from Day One. The Society was founded mainly by clinicians whose clout held sway through the early decades and led to the establishment of JCEM in 1942. My first attendance at an annual meeting was in 1933 in Milwaukee (single room w/b $3.00; double $5.00). There were about 35 registrants, many being prominent clinicians. I distinctly recall lengthy discussions leading off with, "Mr. Chairman, I have a case." Of the 28 papers presented at that meeting 21 were of purely clinical

---

Received February 18, 1991.
* "Remembrance" articles discuss people and events as remembered by the author. The opinion(s) expressed are solely those of the writer and do not reflect the view of the Journal or The Endocrine Society.

nature. I failed to attend a couple of meetings in the late 1940s due to their strong clinical overtones. With the entrance of NIH funding at midcentury and for many years thereafter these meetings came to be predominantly devoted to the interests of basic science investigators. Currently a timely effort is under way to woo back the clinical brethren and achieve a mutually beneficial balance between these two highly overlapping realms of research.

In 1959 while I was on a 6-month sabbatical leave, Ernie Knobil kept the ball rolling smoothly with a daily pilgrimage to the editorial office at my home. This assignment put him in the thick of things which he handled with relish and I think some memorable pleasure.

In the 29 yr since our editorial stint ended I surmise that the present Editor-in-Chief, P. Michael Conn might agree that while much has changed, much remains the same.

Roy O. Greep
Professor Emeritus
Harvard University

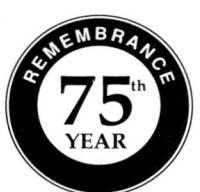

Growth of The Endocrine Society Journals*

The Endocrine Society was organized in 1917 by a pioneering band of 300 charter members for "the advancement, promulgation, and exchange of knowledge regarding the internal secretions." This was to be accomplished via annual meetings and publication of a journal (1). The enterprise has been highly successful. The Endocrine Society, its annual meetings, and its journal publication activities have expanded exponentially since 1917. Society membership in 1990 reached 6333 active members, and annual meeting attendance in 1990 was 4200 persons.

The first journal, Endocrinology, contained 568 pages in its 1917 inaugural year and has grown progressively in yearly pages published to 6472 pages in 1990. In 1952 the Society began publication of a second journal, The Journal of Clinical Endocrinology and Metabolism (JCEM). The JCEM included 1020 pages in 1952 and has grown in yearly published pages to 3494 pages in 1990. Correcting these 1990 page values for a 20% increase in page size (to 8½ by 11 inches in 1979) the 1990 page numbers, in 1978 pages for Endocrinology and JCEM, would be 7766 and 4193, respectively. These data are summarized in Table 1.

As shown in Table I The Endocrine Society now publishes four journals. Endocrine Reviews was inaugurated in 1980 with 435 pages and has expanded modestly in size to 612 pages in 1990. Molecular Endocrinology was introduced in 1987 and started with 950 pages and in 1990 expanded to 2,066 pages. The total text pages published by the Society has increased from 568 in 1917 to 12,644 in 1990; corrected to 1978 pages the 1990 value would be 15,172 pages (Table 1). This latter number represents a 27-fold increase in textual information since 1917. Most of this increase (51%) represents the growth of Endocrinology which now requires four volumes for binding each year.

The history of The Endocrine Society journals reflects the growth of science publications in general. The rate of growth of science literature, in numbers of journals, has been exponential since the 18th century with a doubling time approximating 15 yr (2, 3). The doubling time for the number of Endocrine Society journals approximates 17 yr. The growth of scientific journals has proceeded in parallel with the growth in number of research scientists and has been proposed to represent "a natural consequence of scientific progress" (3). With regard to The Endocrine Society publications, the growth of (corrected) pages published by the Society since 1917 (27-fold) approximates the increase in Society membership (21-fold). This would support the view that the increase in scientific publications correlates with the growth in number of active scientists, in this case, endocrinologists. There has been no important change in the number of pages per journal article, so for The Endocrine Society publications the correlation with active scientists is better for total pages published (27-fold increase vs. 21-fold increase) than for the number of Endocrine Society journals (4-fold increase vs. 21-fold increase).

The quality of The Endocrine Society journals is reflected in Table 2 where data regarding the impact factor, the ratio of journal article citations to the number of articles published as listed in the Institute of Scientific Information (ISI) Science Citation Index, is shown. This index is shown from the first listing in 1975 through 1988 and offers insight into the use of the information by other authors. The number of journals ranked increased from 2434 in 1975 to 4233 in 1988. Both Endocrinology and JCEM consistently rank in the upper 2–4% of the several thousand journals ranked with regard to impact factor. The success of Endocrine Reviews is indicated by its consistent ranking in the top 1% of journals with regard to frequency of citation of published articles. Data are not yet available for Molecular Endocrinology.

The value and significance of the ISI citation data has been questioned, since as many as 50% of papers published are not cited during the 5 yr after publication (4). A variety of reasons for noncitation have been presented to counter the argument that much of the research being done is not worthwhile. Certainly, literature searches are not always careful and comprehensive, self-citation is sometimes overdone, and deliberate exclusion of published work may occur (4). On the other side, some of the published research is redundant and there is a tendency to package research data in least publishable units (LPUs) (5). There are significant correlations of citation frequency with the significance and impact of individual

---

Received March 26, 1991.

* "Remembrance" articles discuss people and events as remembered by the author. The opinion(s) expressed are solely those of the writer and do not reflect the view of the Journal or The Endocrine Society.

TABLE 1. Journal pages published in Endocrine Society Journals 1917–1990[a]

Year	Endocrinology	Journal of Clinical Endocrinology and Metabolism	Endocrine Reviews	Molecular Endocrinology	Total
1917	568				568
1920	714				719
1930	461				461
1940	2,126				2,126
1950	1,069				1,069
1952	1,283	1,020			2,303
1960	1,826	1,683			3,509
1970	2,899	1,520			4,419
1980	4,196	2,667	435		7,298
	(5,035)	(3,200)	(522)		(8,670)
1987	4,917	2,670	500	950	9,037
	(5,903)	(3,204)	(600)	(1,140)	(10,847)
1990	6,472	3,494	612	2066	12,644
	(7,766)	(4,193)	(734)	(2,479)	(15,172)

[a] Numbers in parentheses for 1980 to 1990 represent a correction for comparative purposes for a 20% increase in page size to an 8½ x 11 inch format in 1979.

TABLE 2. Impact factor for Endocrine Society Journals 1975–1988[a]

Year	Endocrinology	Journal of Clinical Endocrinology and Metabolism	Endocrine Reviews	No journals ranked
1975	4,337 (82)	5,170 (53)		2,434
1976	4,700 (58)	5,091 (48)		2,330
1977	4,837 (82)	4,225 (103)		2,730
1978	5,440 (68)	4,072 (121)		3,233
1979	4,728 (89)	4,088 (115)		3,423
1980	4,704 (92)	4,079 (115)		3,536
1981	4,441 (98)	3,685 (140)		3,636
1982	3,767 (159)	3,813 (154)		3,890
1983	4,093 (138)	3,764 (169)	12,152 (15)	3,917
1984	4,347 (115)	3,631 (153)	10,763 (17)	3,910
1985	4,116 (136)	4,213 (130)	9,163 (32)	4,072
1986	4,120 (131)	4,195 (125)	12,976 (16)	4,123
1987	3,839 (152)	4,075 (135)	11,551 (20)	4,159
1988	4,225 (137)	4,091 (145)	10,556 (25)	4,233

[a] Impact factor is the ratio of current year citations of articles published during the previous 2 yr to the number of articles published during the previous 2 yr. The impact factor is listed with the numerical ranking (in parentheses) relative to the total of ranked journals. Data are extracted from the Institute of Scientific Information Science Citation Index.

articles, individual scientists, and individual journals (6–9). These correlations are not perfect for all of the reasons mentioned. Scientists are, in fact, human beings with their share of human foibles. However, notwithstanding the problems and criticisms, there is value, in my view, to the scientific citation databases.

With regard to The Endocrine Society publications, their consistently high citation frequency and "impact factor" coupled with continuing impressive growth indicates that they rank among the important "core journals" of the biological sciences with regard to their quality and effectiveness. The stewards of the Society and its journals and the membership at large can take great satisfaction for their success in continuing to emulate the goals of the society as propounded by the founding fathers—"the advancement, promulgation, and exchange of knowledge regarding the internal secretions."

D. A. Fisher
Professor of Pediatrics
and Medicine
UCLA School of Medicine

References

1. Fisher DA 1984 The Endocrine Society: past and present. J Clin Endocrinol Metab 59:1229–1233
2. Ziman J 1976 The force of knowledge. Cambridge University Press,

3. Ziman JM 1980 The proliferation of scientific literature: a natural process. Science 208:369–371
4. Siekevitz P 1991 Citations and the tenor of the times. FASEB J 5:139
5. Stossel TP 1987 Volume: papers and academic promotion. Ann Intern Med 106:146-148
6. Garfield E 1990 The most cited papers of all time, SCI 1945–1988. Pt 1A, The SCI top 100—Will the Lowry method ever be obliterated? Curr Cont no. 7:3–14
7. Garfield E 1983 How to use citation analysis for faculty evaluations and when is it relevant? Curr Cont no. 44:1–13, no. 45:5–14
8. Garfield E 1978 The 300 most cited authors 1961–1976, including co-authors. Pt 2, The relationship between citedness, awards and academy memberships. Curr Cont no. 35:5–30
9. Garfield E 1987 Why are the impacts of the leading medical journals so similar and yet so different? Item by item audits reveal a diversity of editorial material. Curr Cont no. 2:3–9

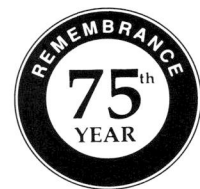

From Enzyme to Transport and back to Enzyme—Insulin Action over Forty Years*

I entered the insulin action field after the hexokinase fiasco in the Cori laboratory. Insulin, added to tissue extracts, supposedly overcame or "deinhibited" hexokinase activity previously inhibited by pituitary extracts or adrenal steroids. This duplicated at the enzyme or hexokinase level the effect of pituitary or adrenal ablation to ameliorate the diabetes of pancreatectomy so elegantly demonstrated by Houssay, Long, and others.

The fraudulent nature of some of the enzyme experiments soon became known. Rachmiel Levine further decimated the hexokinase theory of insulin action with logic and with experiment. He demonstrated, using the eviscerate dog model, that nonutilizable hexoses such as galactose increased in concentration in intracellular water with insulin action. This proved an earlier hypothesis, that insulin increased glucose entry via transport prior to hexokinase action inside the cell. These findings were hotly debated when I was a student in the Cori laboratory, but were soon confirmed by Park and coworkers much to the dismay of the Coris.

I, together with Carlos Villar-Palasi, began investigating insulin action in Earl Sutherland's Department of Pharmacology at Western Reserve University by asking "Does insulin simply increase glucose transport or does the hormone maintain its metabolic interest by directing the glucose intracellularly along certain pathways?" We began to compare on a balance basis, insulin-stimulated glucose uptake to glycogen accumulation. We used the isolated rat diaphragm, a model, it turned out, originally described by Chalmers Gemmill, my immediate predecessor as Chairman of Pharmacology at University of Virginia.

First, we determined the shortest reliable time during which we could quantitatively estimate enhanced glucose uptake and glycogen deposition in the tissue with insulin action. This turned out to be 10 min, then a very short time. Earl Sutherland taught us to do a prior "rundown" period, during which diaphragms were preincubated without hormones (about 30 min) to lower the baseline. We were soon off and running on a jerry-rigged lab bench made up of a piece of plywood placed over two adjoining desks in a medical student laboratory, unused in the summer time. This was the only available lab space in the department.

We rapidly discovered that better than 90% of the insulin-stimulated glucose uptake from the medium was accounted for by glycogen accumulation in the tissue. This was an extraordinarily high yield, approaching theoretical when the extra glucose oxidized was calculated in. This high yield was not duplicated by increasing the glucose concentration in the medium without insulin added.

To get at the mechanism, we next systematically measured all the known tissue intermediates between glucose and glycogen and the high energy phosphates as well. No changes were seen in ATP, ADP, AMP, P_i, or creatine phosphate. However, glucose 6-P was increased with insulin action, as would have been expected from increased transport. But to our surprize, the next known intermediate toward glycogen, glucose 1-P was not increased even in the face of a major increase in glycogen. Quantitative determination of glucose 1-P was novel in the literature at that time, taking a good deal of ingenuity on our part to achieve. It was a pivotal measurement for two reasons; first, located between glucose 6-P and glycogen, it should have been increased by the push provided by increased transport. But it was not. We therefore suggested that in addition to transport, insulin acted intracellularly to exert a "pull" between glucose 1-P and glycogen. This was heretical. Second, and of equal importance, the quantitative estimation of glucose 1-P and P_i allowed us to calculate ratios of glucose 1-P/P_i which were compared to the well known equilibrium ratio for the enzyme phosphorylase, thought to be responsible for glycogen synthesis based on the work of the Coris. They had recently received the Nobel Prize for their elucidation of the action of this enzyme and its ability to catalyze the synthesis of a glycogen-like polysaccharide in a test tube in the presence of a glycogen primer.

However, the equilibrium ratios which we calculated from our experiments were 75- to 100-fold removed from the phosphorylase equilibrium and were in the direction of glycogen degradation. In simple terms, P_i was present in much too high a concentration to ever allow synthesis

---

Received February 14, 1991.

* "Remembrance" articles discuss people and events as remembered by the author. The opinion(s) expressed are solely those of the writer and do not reflect the view of the Journal or The Endocrine Society.

of glycogen by phosphorylase. We therefore began to seriously consider and propose a new pathway for glycogen synthesis bypassing P_i.

Just at this time, Leloir and Cardini published a brief note describing a very weak enzyme activity in liver extracts which catalyzed the direct transfer of glucose from UDPG to glycogen. We rapidly confirmed this finding in muscle extracts, the insulin-sensitive tissue of our interest. We also demonstrated that the equilibrium of the new enzyme reaction was essentially totally displaced in the direction of glycogen synthesis in contrast to phosphorylase which was readily reversible. We further demonstrated the presence in muscle extracts of the enzyme catalyzing the synthesis of UDPG from UTP and glucose 1-P, namely UDPG pyrophosphorylase. At that time this enzyme had only been identified in yeast by Kalckar and co-workers.

These two new enzymes coupled together forming a pathway for glycogen synthesis which proceeded through PP_i and bypassed P_i. This fit our criteria and, in addition, fit a proposal by Kornberg that enzymes catalyzing biosynthetic reaction pathways, in general, went via PP_i, while degradative reactions were catalyzed by enzymes via P_i. This logically meant that phosphorylase catalyzed glycogen degradation in the cell, while the two new enzymes catalyzed synthesis. We proposed a glycogen cycle comprising both biosynthetic and degradative reactions. This concept has stood the test of time and recently direct evidence for glycogen cycling has been obtained with nuclear magnetic resonance technology.

You can imagine what a stir this data and interpretation caused. The mechanism of insulin action was enhanced glucose transport. Our papers were all turned down by the *Journal of Biological Chemistry* with sincere apologies, and subsequently published in *Archives of Biochemistry and Biophysics*. Carl Cori would never accept the synthetic role for the new pathway until years later when a patient with McArdle's disease, muscle phosphorylase deficiency, had glycogen storage together with the two new enzymes of glycogen synthesis present. Rachmiel Levine at that time vigorously opposed the work and interpretation. But to his great credit, Rachmiel has subsequently publically stated his support and admiration for the work. In fact, it explained some of his own earlier published data on glycogen accumulation with insulin in the eviscerate dog model which he had not understood and to which he had paid little attention since it had not fit neatly into the increased transport mechanism.

Having identified four enzymes, two old, phosphorylase and phosphoglucomutase, and two new, UDPG pyrophosphorylase, and glycogen synthase comprising the glycogen cycle, we next "took the bull by the horns" and decided to directly measure their activities after insulin treatment. We knew from our hexose-P measurements that glucose 6-P was increased in the insulin-treated tissue whereas glucose 1-P was not. We reasoned therefore, that either the UDPG pyrophosphorylase or the glycogen synthase step might be activated by insulin. It was also theoretically possible that phosphorylase or phosphoglucomutase might be affected.

We had one crucial additional fact to go on; namely, the report from Leloir's lab that glucose 6-P activated glycogen synthase in the test tube. We had already confirmed this in our lab and found that the concentration dependence was in the range of our tissue concentrations. We therefore decided that in order to determine whether glucose 6-P was in fact stimulating glycogen synthase to synthesize glycogen in insulin-stimulated muscle, we would assay the enzyme in two ways. First, we would assay the enzyme with no additions to detect the increased enzyme activity due to the increased glucose 6-P in the extract from the insulin-treated tissue. Second, we would add excess glucose 6-P to fully saturate and fully stimulate the enzyme to its maximal activity. Under these conditions we would not expect to find any difference between the control and insulin extracts. This so called plus-minus assay was modeled after the phosphorylase assay done with and without adenylic acid to detect active *a* form and total enzyme activity (sum of active and inactive forms).

We were very excited to see the anticipated result after the first experiment, namely minus glucose 6-P, a 30% increase in the glycogen synthase activity in the insulin extract compared to control. With added glucose 6-P, no difference was seen in the "total" enzyme activity. When the other three enzymes were assayed, no differences were seen. Of the four enzymes, glycogen synthase activity was lowest, and rate limiting, phosphoglucomutase was highest, and the others of intermediate activity.

We next set out to prove that glucose 6-P was the activating factor in the extracts. However, calculations soon showed that in the diluted reaction mixtures, the glucose 6-P concentrations were too low to stimulate glycogen synthase.

To definitively rule glucose 6-P in or out, we did several experiments to determine whether the increased glycogen synthase seen with insulin treatment remained or was lost after glucose 6-P was removed. We dialyzed the enzyme, and we precipitated it with ammonium sulfate. Both techniques told us that when we removed the glucose 6-P, the increased enzyme activity with insulin remained. It was a stable effect, not explained by the presence of glucose 6-P. Tightly bound glucose 6-P was ruled out by adding excess glucose 6-P to the extracts and removing it by ammonium sulfate precipitation of the enzyme, washing the precipitated enzyme, redissolving it, and recovering the original nonstimulated enzyme activity.

Our data now suggested that the cause of the increased enzyme activity was not increased glucose 6-P, but rather a stable change in the enzyme. Further, since there was no change in the total activity, insulin had apparently acted to convert an inactive form of the enzyme to an active form. This is what the assay had detected even though it had been designed to detect an increase in a soluble activator. Two forms of the enzyme were accordingly proposed, in analogy with phosphorylase, an active or "independent" form which did not require glucose 6-P, and an inactive or "dependent" form which absolutely required glucose 6-P for activity.

We immediately began purifying the enzyme, always assaying with the plus-minus assay looking for ways to separate the two forms. We found wide variations in activity ratios depending on tissues, species, and types of preparations. The early results were encouraging. For example, early studies of frog and toadfish muscle revealed only the inactive or dependent form. Ratios of activity in rat muscle were variable depending on conditions. When rat muscle extracts were incubated in mercaptoethanol to test stability, the enzyme became converted from a mixture of active and inactive forms, to an essentially totally active form. Alternatively, when ATP was added to check the effects of nucleotides, the enzyme was inhibited. We soon determined that the inhibition was a stable one, and that the inhibited inactive form of the enzyme could be purified and characterized kinetically. The effect of glucose 6-P was to markedly increase Vm. Similarly, the active form from rat muscle was purified and characterized kinetically. The effect of glucose 6-P was small, and resulted in a slight decrease in Michaelis-Menten constant (K_m). These early studies were done with Carlos Villar-Palasi and the late Manolo Rosell-Perez.

Dan Friedman, a graduate student and I next went on to work out the biochemical basis of the stability of the two forms and of the two interconversion reactions. We were fortunate in having the interconversions of phosphorylase as a model to go on. We soon discovered that [^{32}P] from [^{32}P]ATP was incorporated into the enzyme with conversion of the active to inactive form. Conversely, [^{32}P] was released from the enzyme when it became activated. Dan went on to purify the kinase, separating it from phosphorylase b kinase. With Frans Huijing, we demonstrated that it was stimulated by cAMP in the micromolar range. This was the first demonstration of the cAMP kinase, called, at that time, glycogen synthase kinase. Krebs and co-workers used our purification proceedure to identify the same enzyme which they called phosphorylase b kinase kinase. The Krebs group found that the new kinase acted on commercially available histone and casein substrates and renamed the enzyme cAMP-dependent protein kinase.

This was the beginning of our search for the mechanism of insulin action. A search for insulin's effect on the cAMP-dependent protein kinase led to the discovery of its inactivation by insulin treatment. This in turn led to development of an assay for the putative insulin mediator, which, in turn has led to the isolation of two separate phosphoinositol glycan species of mediator containing two separate inositol species.

What is fascinating to consider is the new knowledge that has come from studies of the insulin receptor. Upon binding of the hormone, an early, if not the initial event, is activation of the tyrosine kinase enzyme in the receptor B chain. Binding of the hormone transmits a steric signal which directly activates the enzyme. So, we have come a full circle in our thinking. From the hormone activating hexokinase, an intracellular enzyme, to its acting on the antecedant transport step, back to its acting directly on an enzyme in the receptor itself. It is now recognized that a cascade of dephosphorylations and increased phosphorylations ensue from this initial event which include the dephosphorylation of glycogen synthase the first discovered, and then pyruvate dehydrogenase, activating these rate-limiting steps in glycogen and fat synthesis. The insulin mediators which are also formed coupled to receptor occupancy, presumably act to regulate this cascade by controlling the activity of several kinases and phosphatases.

I think that after many false starts, we are now on the right track to understand insulin's action, now renamed signalling. Insulin action has always been difficult to understand because insulin is a "maverick" employing several parallel different signalling mechanisms simultaneously rather than one. The human mind would much prefer to have one.

Joseph Larner
Professor of Pharmacology
University of Virginia

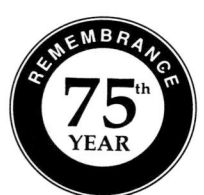

Remembrances of the Meadowbrook Conferences—When Steroids Came to DNA

The majestic, manorial ambience of Meadowbrook Hall—a 51-room Tudor mansion in a park-like setting amid the rolling hills of Michigan—seems an appropriate metaphor for the splendid conceptual developments in steroid hormone action that have unfolded during the last decade. With the first availability of recombinant DNA technology for endocrinological investigation, we all felt a pleasant tension of excitement and anticipation—certain that something more than ambiguous conclusions based on an endless array of sucrose gradient peaks was about to emerge. Many long-time workers in the field experienced a less pleasant, albeit needless, tension as well: the fear that "retooling" for the new technology would prove an insurmountable difficulty and that the entire field in which they had labored so long would be engulfed by the domain of microbiology and virology. The previous two decades had seen the rise and fall of two well publicized dogmas: Paul Talalay's transhydrogenation model and Gordon Tomkins' posttranscription model. Would Elwood Jensen's two-step receptor model, combined with Bert O'Malley's massive assault on the ovalbumin gene, provide the right answer?

In the midst of this uncertain period in the history of endocrinology, we organized the first Meadowbrook Conference on Steroid Hormone Action. Since that first conference in the fall of 1978, almost all of the major laborers in the vineyard of endocrinology have had at least one opportunity to enjoy a temporary baronial existence within the elegant walls of Meadowbrook Hall.

At the first conference, it became clear that Bert O'Malley was engaged in exploiting the emergent techniques of molecular biology to their limit with his ovalbumin model. Newly created immigrants from other territories in the field were searching diligently for appropriate, hopefully better models that would use the new techniques to unravel the mystery of hormone action. There was a general consensus among the members of the molecular biology community that the mechanism of eukaryotic gene regulation might not be too different from that of the bacterial operons. Where then would be a better place to start than the steroid (lactose), receptor (repressor) and the target gene (operon)? Everyone was keenly aware that, two decades earlier, the appropriate choice of model had played a key role in the historic success of Jacob and Monod. Robert Goldberger, formerly a prokaryotic biologist, began his presentation with a justification for his choice of estrogenic regulation of vitellogenin in the chicken liver as the model for exploring the molecular basis of steroid hormone action. Hoping it would be a better model, and perhaps less complicated, than ovalbumin, he outlined five questions: "Where can I find a system which 1) responds exclusively to a steroid hormone [and] 2) produces a large amount of the induced protein [in which] 3) the responsive tissue provides an adequate mass with homogeneous cell population, 4) the tissue contains well characterized estrogen receptor, and 5) differentiation is not involved in hormone response." He then went on to describe his elegant studies on estrogenic regulation of vitellogenin gene expression in the avian liver. After he finished, William Schrader stood up with a grin on his face and, in his characteristic way, said, "Bob, you asked about finding a model where no differentiation was involved and what not. My question is, to whom did you address these questions and how was the answer forthcoming? My next question is, in a less ecclesiastical vein ..." The whole room exploded into laughter.

Besides some of these lighter moments, the first conference saw the resolution of many serious matters and the emergence of new ideas. Except for a very few brave souls, most of the endocrinologists during that time were not conceptually ready to expect the inevitable: direct receptor-DNA interactions as the molecular basis of target gene induction. They remained preoccupied with alternative possibilities; clearly, an in-depth soul searching was in order. Out of this morass of new considerations were to emerge ideas later shown to be prophetic. For example, Gerald Mueller, in his introductory remarks, commented that steroid receptors are always found in association with other proteins. "The proteins in these receptor complexes have been disregarded for too long," he said. "We need to establish their identity." Discovery of the association and role of heat shock proteins in steroid receptor function in the laboratories of Etienne

---

Received February 12, 1991.
"Remembrance" articles discuss people and events as remembered by the author. The opinion(s) expressed are solely those of the writer and do not reflect the view of the Journal or The Endocrine Society.

Baulieu, Bill Pratt, David Toft, and others has subsequently lent substance to the visionary comments made by Gerry back in 1978.

The second conference was held in the fall of 1981—a time when endocrinology, and especially the area of steroid hormone action, had come to a crossroads and new tools of recombinant DNA technology had already begun to make their mark. Not only was the dynamics of steroid-receptor interaction and subsequent receptor migration into the nucleus being hotly debated, the complexity of the eukaryotic chromatin structure continued to frustrate the regulon modelers. Relief was to come from an unexpected source, outside the big-time ovalbumin and vitellogenin gene explorers. Keith Yamamoto in San Francisco and Jan Ake Gustafsson in Sweden firmed up a long-distance collaboration: Jan Ake with his large team of co-workers in Huddinge would purify the needed amount of glucocorticoid receptor and Keith, with his smaller group, would examine specific binding of the receptor to various fragments of the murine mammary tumor virus (MMTV), whose expression was known to be regulated by glucocorticoids. Although similar experiments with purified progesterone receptor and fragments of the ovalbumin gene had previously supplied disappointing results, the MMTV-glucocorticoid receptor system, in the hands of these investigators, provided a historic breakthrough. Jan Ake's results were received with more than a moderate degree of skepticism—and he demonstrated some reluctance to divulge everything that he had in mind. The mood of that evening was caught in this exchange between John Anderson and Jan Ake Gustafsson.

Anderson: "Wouldn't you expect that, if indeed there is specific binding, the calf thymus DNA would give some competitive effect because the DNA would be expected to have some glucocorticoid binding sites?"
Gustafsson: "These results will be described in detail in the forthcoming PNAS paper."
Anderson: "Wasn't it said in the paper that 10,000-fold excess of calf thymus DNA did not exhibit competition?"
Gustafsson: "No, but if you wait another month, you will see the PNAS paper and you can check that."

Soon thereafter, everything came out in print and the rest is history. We know today that there is basically very little difference between pro- and eukaryotic regulons. The signal transducers, *i.e.* the receptor proteins, interact with the response elements defined by a short segment of DNA on the target gene, and endocrinologists can rightfully claim the credit for this historical development in regulatory biology. Space and the delicacy of social circumspection do not permit me to describe all the many colorful social events that transpired during the second conference or the many interesting anecdotes resulting therefrom, but rest assured that I will pass them on to my students and friends, thus preserving them for posterity. However, one important scientific tidbit dare not go unmentioned, because of its historic significance. Brad Thompson, after a significant dose of liquid refreshment, took microphone in hand and adopted the role of soothsayer: "I suggest that receptors are going to be a multigene family in which the steroid binding site is relatively constant.... On the other hand, the DNA-binding regions are separated by a widely variable set of sequences in the genomic DNA." This statement did indeed have a prophetic ring. One has to remember that this was in 1981—long before any receptor gene had been cloned or its sequence deciphered.

By 1981, the course of the field had been irreversibly set and the two subsequent conferences, held in 1985 and 1988, witnessed the identification of steroid response elements in almost all of the target genes, hormone-dependent expression of the promoter-reporter constructs in the transfected cells and cell-free systems and, above all, cloning of the genes of various steroid receptors.

It is testimony to the leadership, imagination and dexterity of endocrinologists that we have been able to attain an understanding of eukaryotic gene regulation to the level of the *Escherichia coli* operon within only 20 yr, considering the enormous differences in order of complexity between the *E. coli* and the vertebrate genome. The next 20 yr promises to be at least equally exciting, and perhaps more so, due to the convergence of regulatory mechanisms involving hormone receptors, oncogenes, and growth factors. The "Brave New World" on whose border we stood in 1978 is no longer an alien territory, but a charted landscape, whose features we continue to define and explore with more anticipation than trepidation.

Arun K. Roy
Division of Molecular Genetics
Department of Obstetrics/Gynecology
University of Texas Health Science Center

Remembrances of Contributions of Philip Smith and Bernardo Houssay to the Development of Neuroendocrinology

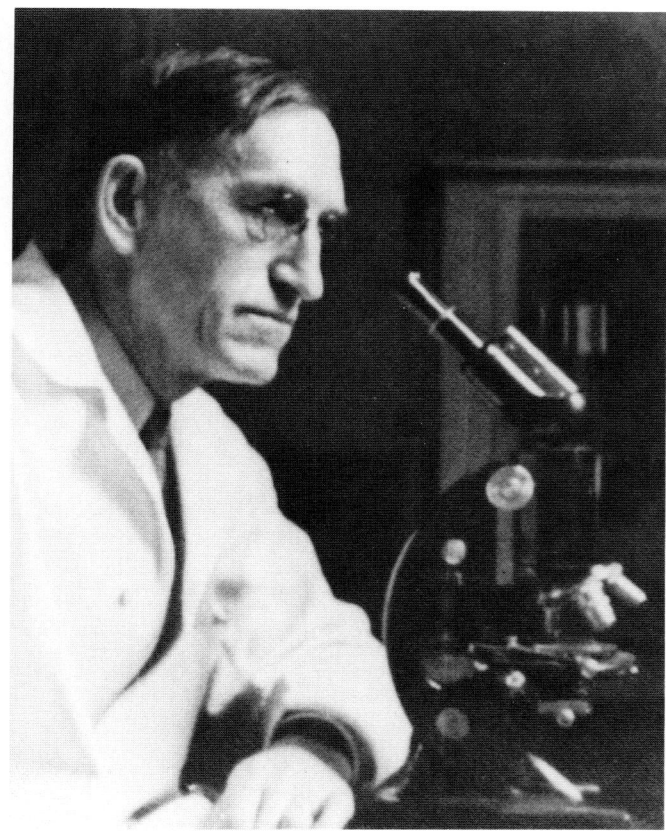
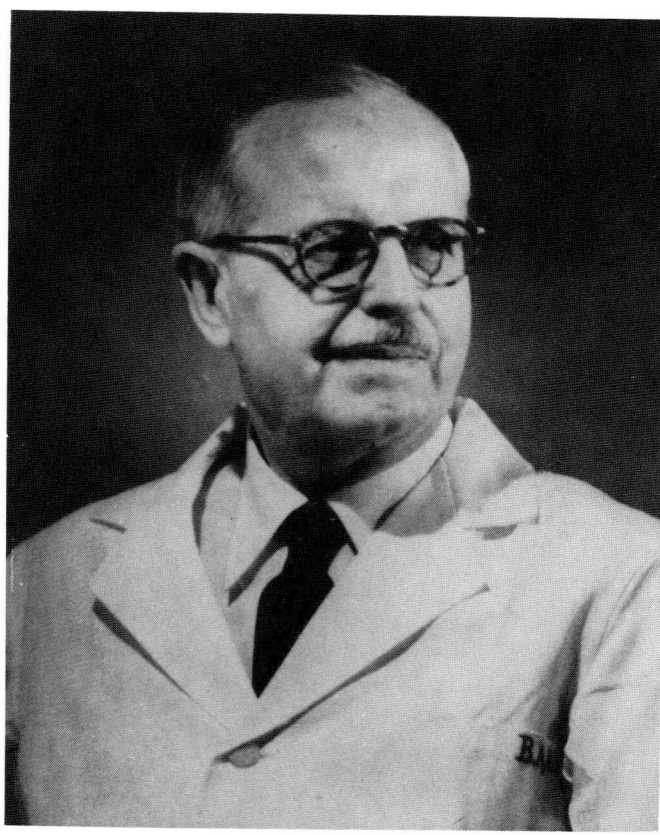

FIG. 1. *Left*, Philip E. Smith (1884–1970). *Right*, Bernardo A. Houssay (1887–1971). From: Ref. 1, page 26. (Courtesy of the American Physiological Society).

Two endocrinologists whose work I always greatly admired, starting in my early graduate student days, and whom I later came to know personally were Philip Smith and Bernardo Houssay. Although both have been universally esteemed and honored as preeminent endocrinologists, their pioneer efforts in neuroendocrinology have not always been recognized as such. Both exerted tremendous influence not only from the importance of their own research, but also because of the many students they trained. Both possessed warm, modest, friendly personalities and were happy to discuss the work of younger colleagues with them. Both lived well past their 80th birthdays, but died in the early 1970s, too early to prepare a chapter for the 1975 volume of *Pioneers in Neuroendocrinology*.

A major component of Smith's success lay in his remarkable ability to devise and execute precise techniques for clean hypophysectomy that did not damage the hypothalamus. Starting 75 yr ago at the University of California at Berkeley, he developed and published a

Received March 12, 1991.
"Remembrance" articles discuss people and events as remembered by the author. The opinion(s) expressed are solely those of the writer and do not reflect the view of the Journal or The Endocrine Society.

method of hypophysectomizing frog embryos by removing the buccal anlage. Later at Berkeley, Stanford, and Columbia, he became the world's authority on parapharyngeal hypophysectomy techniques in mammals, devising successively methods for rats, rabbits, dogs, and monkeys. With his expertise in rats, in 1930 he published his classic study on "hypophysectomy and replacement therapy" in which he showed conclusively that the pituitary gland produced hormones regulating growth, adrenals, thyroid, and gonads. With clean hypophysectomy there was no tendency toward the adiposity characteristic of Fröhlich's adiposogenital syndrome. He induced the latter by intrapituitary injections of chromic acid via a temporal approach, undoubtedly attributable to hypothalamic damage. He next used clean parapharyngeal hypophysectomy in the reflexly ovulating rabbit to extend the 1929 findings of Fee and Parkes that an ovulatory quantum of pituitary gonadotropin was released as a neuroendocrine response to the coital stimulus within an hour after mating; he added that in the absence of the hypophysis the new corpora lutea were not maintained. Developing an interest in the hypothalamo-pituitary portal system at the time of his retirement from Columbia, Smith returned to Stanford as an emeritus research associate in his late 70s and published his final important studies on the complete recovery of pituitary function in rats, hypophysectomized several months earlier, by implanting young pituitaries under the median eminence where portal veins could reach them by regeneration. Implants to other sites did not restore function.

Houssay was more neurally oriented than Smith. His early experiments were also with an amphibian, the argentine toad *Bufo arenarum*. He found that purely hypothalamic lesions inhibited sexual behavior. Infundibulohypophyseal lesions made with a hot needle caused a central infarct in adenohypophyseal circulation, resulting in polyuria and deficiencies in gonadal, thyroid, and pancreatic function. These were induced by damage to the pituitary portal system which arose in the infundibular lobe and flowed toward the principal lobe; the deficiencies were corrected as the portal vessels regenerated. The 1935 paper describing the direction of portal flow as seen in the living toad had an interesting history: published in the French Comptes Rendus des Seances, a year before the appearance of Wislocki and King's histological studies of the portal system, it became completely lost in the literature and was never quoted. It was finally resurrected and cited 12 yr later by Green in 1947, only after he had independently made a similar observation in the living frog. In the meantime Houssay's fame from his research on the role of the hypophysis in carbohydrate metabolism and diabetes performed on many mammals, especially dogs, as well as on toads, had won him the Nobel Prize in Physiology and Medicine in 1947. In addition to more than 500 research publications and several books, Houssay also contributed an important textbook of physiology which was outstanding in its coverage of endocrine secretion.

I am happy to have had the privilege of recalling these incidents in the development of neuroendocrinology, literature references to which may be found in the essay (1).

Charles H. Sawyer
Department of Anatomy and Cell Biology
University of California—Los Angeles
School of Medicine

References

1. Sawyer CH Anterior pituitary neural control concepts. In: Endocrinology: People and Ideas, McCann SM (ed) American Physiological Society, Bethesda, MD, 1988, chap 2, pp 23–39

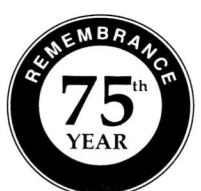

Glycoprotein Hormones Were Always Composed of Subunits—We Just Had to Find Out the Hard Way

The glycoprotein hormones of the pituitary gland (LH, FSH, and TSH) each consist of two chemically dissimilar, dissociable, glycosylated protein subunits. One of the subunits (α) is common and identical in primary structure in all three hormones; the other (β) determines the hormone specificity of the fully active α-β complex. The chorionic gonadotropins (human CG, equine CG) have a similar chemistry. Over the last 20 yr this basic description has appeared so many times in papers on glycoprotein hormones that the source references are no longer cited. *i.e.* it is now dogma. This, of course, is very aggravating to those of my generation that played a role in developing the above concepts. Since it may seem odd to our younger colleagues that the subunit nature of the glycoprotein hormones was not forever evident, and since few of us read scientific papers that are older than 5 yr other than our own masterpieces, I would like to briefly cover in this "Remembrance" those key studies that led in a matter of a few years to a radically new understanding of the structure-function relationships among the glycoprotein hormones. My recollections are highly biased, and I apologize in advance to those whose work I do not mention, especially when they are good friends.

Ovine LH (oLH) was the first of the pituitary and placental glycoprotein hormones in which the subunit nature as described above was demonstrated. By 1959 two laboratories (P. G. Squire in C. H. Li's laboratory in Berkeley and D. N. Ward in Houston) had isolated oLH in a state of purity such that chemical characterization studies could be undertaken. There was reasonable agreement between the two laboratories with respect to such properties as biological potency, amino acid composition, and mol wt, the latter being 28–30,000. In general, all investigators working with gonadotropins or TSH in this period were plagued by problems of low yields, capricious losses of activity, and evidences of polymorphism such that there was difficulty if not reluctance in performing major chemical studies such as amino acid sequencing.

My own work with gonadotropins and oLH in particular began after a year (1961–1962) as a Fellow in Professor Albert Neuberger's laboratory at St. Mary's Hospital in London where I participated in studies on the nature of the carbohydrate-protein linkage in ovalbumin and ovomucoid. Upon my return to Berkeley it seemed sensible to perform similar studies on oLH (or ICSH, interstitial cell-stimulating hormone as it was called in Li's laboratory). I was appalled, however, at the few milligrams of oLH that Dr. Li gave me for a year's study as I had been accustomed to working with gram quantities of the egg white proteins. Using proteolytic digestions, gel filtration, and some semiquantitative carbohydrate analyses, I was able to publish a note in 1963 in *Biophys Biochim Acta* and prepare an abstract for the 1964 Endocrine Society Meeting which concluded that there were two carbohydrate moieties associated with oLH.

It was during this period that perhaps the most important observation relating to the chemistry of oLH and subsequently the other glycoprotein hormones was made by C. H. Li and his research assistant at the time, Barbra Starman. They had been examining the molecular weights of several of the purified pituitary hormones available at that time by the technique of sedimentation-equillibrium, a procedure which had become possible because of advances in ultracentrifuge technology. When they examined oLH in strongly acidic solutions (pH 1.3) they were surprised to find that the mol wt was no longer 30,000 as in neutral solutions but, instead, about 16,000, or roughly half. These results were published as a very short article that appeared in *Nature* in 1964 in which determination of the "monomer" mol wt of ICSH (LH) was described. There was no reason to believe at the time that this was anything but a dimer-monomer dissociation phenomenon. Darrell Ward confirmed and extended the observation the following year (1965) in an article in *Analytical Biochemistry*.

A year later (1966) in an abstract presented at the Federation Meetings Darrell Ward presented data on the amino acid sequences associated with two glycopeptides isolated from proteolytic digests of oLH. These were different and he correctly postulated that the "monomer" chains of oLH were not identical. I had reached the same conclusion from examining tryptic digests of performic acid oxidized oLH by two dimensional chromatography-

---

Received March 18, 1991.

"Remembrance" articles discuss people and events as remembered by the author. The opinion(s) expressed are solely those of the writer and do not reflect the view of the Journal or The Endocrine Society.

electrophoresis on paper. If oLH was a monomer of 15,000 daltons it would have a lysine and arginine content such that one would expect to observe a maximum of about 12 tryptic peptides. Over twice that number was observed suggesting that the units were different but each of about the same mol wt. Additionally, I found that performic acid oxidized preparations of oLH were partially insoluble at pH 4.0 and the two fractions had very different amino acid compositions. Such materials, however, while useful for chemical studies, could not be employed for biological work, and I decided to look for a means of obtaining intact subunits.

I opted for counter-current distribution (CCD) because C. H. Li's laboratory had previously made extensive use of the technique in studies on MSH, ACTH, and PRL. I had used it as well a few years earlier in the purification of porcine GH. Success would depend on finding a two-phase solvent system in which the subunits would differentially partition. Most of the dozen or more organic alcohol-water systems we tried were complete failures in that none of the LH would distribute into the organic phase. One system, however, showed a glimmer of promise. This consisted of 40% ammonium sulfate solution and ethanol and had been tried unsuccessfully by Denis Gospodarowicz a couple of years previously when he worked with me in developing new purification methods for oLH and FSH. By trial and error the system was modified by the addition of dichloroacetic acid to provide an acidic dissociating environment and the introduction of n-propanol in addition to the ethanol as it increased solubility in the organic phase. A limited test of a few transfers with a few milligrams of LH showed great promise and we were ready to try a scaled up experiment with a larger quantity of LH.

However, it was now late in 1966 and we had to suspend our research activity in Berkeley to prepare for our move to San Francisco. December was spent packing and January of 1967 was spent moving and unpacking. As with all such moves the new laboratory was chaos. At the beginning of February, with a minimum of functional equipment, we reinitiated our CCD studies of oLH. Our first experiment which involved 10–20 mg LH and only nine transfers was a spectacular success. The LH had distributed itself into two nearly equal fractions, one of which had a very low partition coefficient and was found mainly in the initial aqueous phases, and one which had a very high partition coefficient which had distributed into the organic phases at the end of the train. We soon had two fractions (called C-I and C-II at that time) which were chemically and electrophoretically different, each of minimal biological activity (about 7% that of intact oLH), and upon mixing and incubating together, a significant regeneration of activity (about 20%) occurred. Indeed we had separated and isolated the subunits of oLH! By early May 1967, Dr. T. S. A. Samy (now at University of Miami School of Medicine) and I submitted a short paper on the preparation and characterization of the subunits of oLH to a well known weekly scientific journal in the US. Needless to say, it was rejected, but happily, was published in another journal several months later (Biochim Biophys Acta 147:175–177, 1967). Earlier in the year Marian Jutisz and his colleagues in Paris published studies in *Biochem Biophys Res Commun* on the dissociation of oLH in concentrated urea solutions, an approach that was later coupled with ion exchange chromatography and used extensively to dissociate and isolate the human pituitary glycoprotein hormone subunits as well as those of human CG and equine CG.

Some of the elegant and now classic studies of John G. Pierce on the chemistry of bovine TSH are necessary to complete this story. While all of the above was taking place, John had decided to ignore the polymorphism of his TSH preparations and proceed with a major effort of determining its amino acid sequence. Despite the convincing evidence of subunits in oLH, similar experiments, including CCD, did not provide such evidence for TSH. On the other hand he found that the amino acid sequences of two of the three glycopeptides of TSH were identical to those of oLH reported by Darrell Ward at the Third International Congress of Endocrinology in 1968, suggesting a close similarity to oLH (J Biol Chem 1969). The big breakthrough came from a serendiptitious set of conditions which, according to John Pierce in his Eli Lilly Lecture in 1971, "allowed the subunits of TSH to more or less fall into our laps." John had found that if TSH were incubated in 1 M propionic acid, lyophilized, and then gel filtered on a column of Sephadex G100 in ammonium bicarbonate, three peaks were eluted which proved to be undissociated TSH, TSH-a, and TSH-b (Federation Meetings 1970). We (Papkoff and Ekblad) later found the same procedure to be applicable to preparing subunits from ovine FSH. John Pierce's progress was now rapid. In comparing the TSH subunits with those of bovine LH prepared by CCD, he showed that one of them (α) was common and interchangeable with respect to generating biological activity and that their tryptic peptides were identical (J Biol Chem 1970, 1971). Thus, all of the essential elements of the subunit nature of the glycoprotein hormones had been demonstrated in a matter of 4 yr after the separation and isolation of the oLH subunits in 1967.

The reader may be interested in the origin of the α-β nomenclature for the subunits of the glycoprotein hormones. It was clear by early 1970 that we were headed for a good deal of confusion as already a half dozen investigators were using different designations for subunits of a particular species of glycoprotein hormone. John Pierce and I must have been very concerned by this because we sent a joint letter dated August 13, 1970 to about 30 investigators in the field throughout the world proposing the α-β nomenclature. In addition, John reiterated the proposal when he gave his landmark presentation on TSH a couple of weeks later at the Laurentian Hormone Conference. There was an immediate acceptance on the part of everyone, possibly because it made sense, but more likely because nobody had to adopt the designations of someone else at the expense of their own nomenclature.

Harold Papkoff
Hormone Research Institute
San Francisco, California

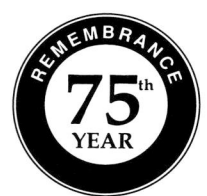

Origin of the Hormone Action Gordon Research Conference

Like a pearl, the Hormone Action Conference began as a result of an irritation. In the summer of 1967, I was invited to give the first talk (on methods to measure protein and nucleic acid synthesis rates, what was called "molecular biology" in those days) at a Gordon Conference that I won't specify for obvious reasons. As the week progressed, I found that the program was not one very close to my own interests and experience; in short, I got pretty bored. So my mind wandered back to a Gatlinberg Conference on effects of hormones a few years earlier (organized, I think, by Frank Kenney), and I wondered why something like that wasn't offered on the Gordon Conference program. Certainly that would be much more interesting, at least from my point of view.

Then as now it was customary for the Executive Director of the GRCs to visit each meeting site each week. In contrast to popular belief, Alex Cruickshank has not been Executive Director since the Conferences first started in 1931. In fact, it was Alex's predecessor, George Park, who visited the Tilton School that week. When I asked him why there was no Conference on Endocrinology, he suggested that I submit a proposal for one. My response that I was by no means a major leader in the field didn't bother him; his reply was to the effect that somebody has to get these things going. (The GRC organization takes a somewhat different view in 1991.) So he sent the forms, and I had a wonderful time putting together a program for the meeting that I personally most wanted to hear. It seemed to me that the most interesting part of Endocrinology then and in the forseeable future was shifting from isolation and chemical characterization of hormones to mechanistic studies of their effects, so I chose "Hormone Action" as the title of the Conference. For a long time, there was no response to the application, and I nearly forgot about the whole thing. Finally I returned from a trip in September 1968 and found a phone message that my application for a Hormone Action Gordon Research Conference had been approved, and I should have a final program ready by January 1 for publication in Science in March.

Fortunately for me, and even more so for the Conference, the field was developing rapidly and had lots of inherent strength, because I did virtually everything wrong. It didn't even occur to me to submit an application to NIH or NSF for support; after all, I had the Chairman's Fund (then $5000) to support speakers. Except for Jay Tepperman (located at the neighboring SUNY Upstate Medical Center), I didn't contact a lot of other people for advice on the program; I just put together the one I most wanted to hear. Assuming that there would be a reasonable number of refusals, I invited more speakers than I really intended to have on the program, and did the entire thing by letter, not phoning anyone (as I recall). I was astonished that only one person declined to appear on the program; his flimsy excuse was that he had been invited to a meeting in Switzerland that week. So I started my association with the Gordon Conferences by doing something I have subsequently criticized a lot of other people for doing, scheduling too many speakers in some sessions. This was back in the days before posters, and I decided to try to keep things open for late-breaking stuff by having FASEB-like short talks during one entire evening session. This was not a big success, to say the least, and it would have horrified my current colleagues on the GRC Board of Trustees.

But it seems that the Conference as a whole was a success. At least, it has certainly lasted a long time, and remained lively and active for more than 20 years now. The poem by Frances Finn, which follows this, chronicles events since that first Conference in 1969.

James R. Florini
Biology Department
Syracuse University

Received May 2, 1991.
"Remembrance," articles discuss people and events as remembered by the author. The opinion(s) expressed are solely those of the writer and do not reflect the view of the Journal or The Endocrine Society.

REMEMBRANCE

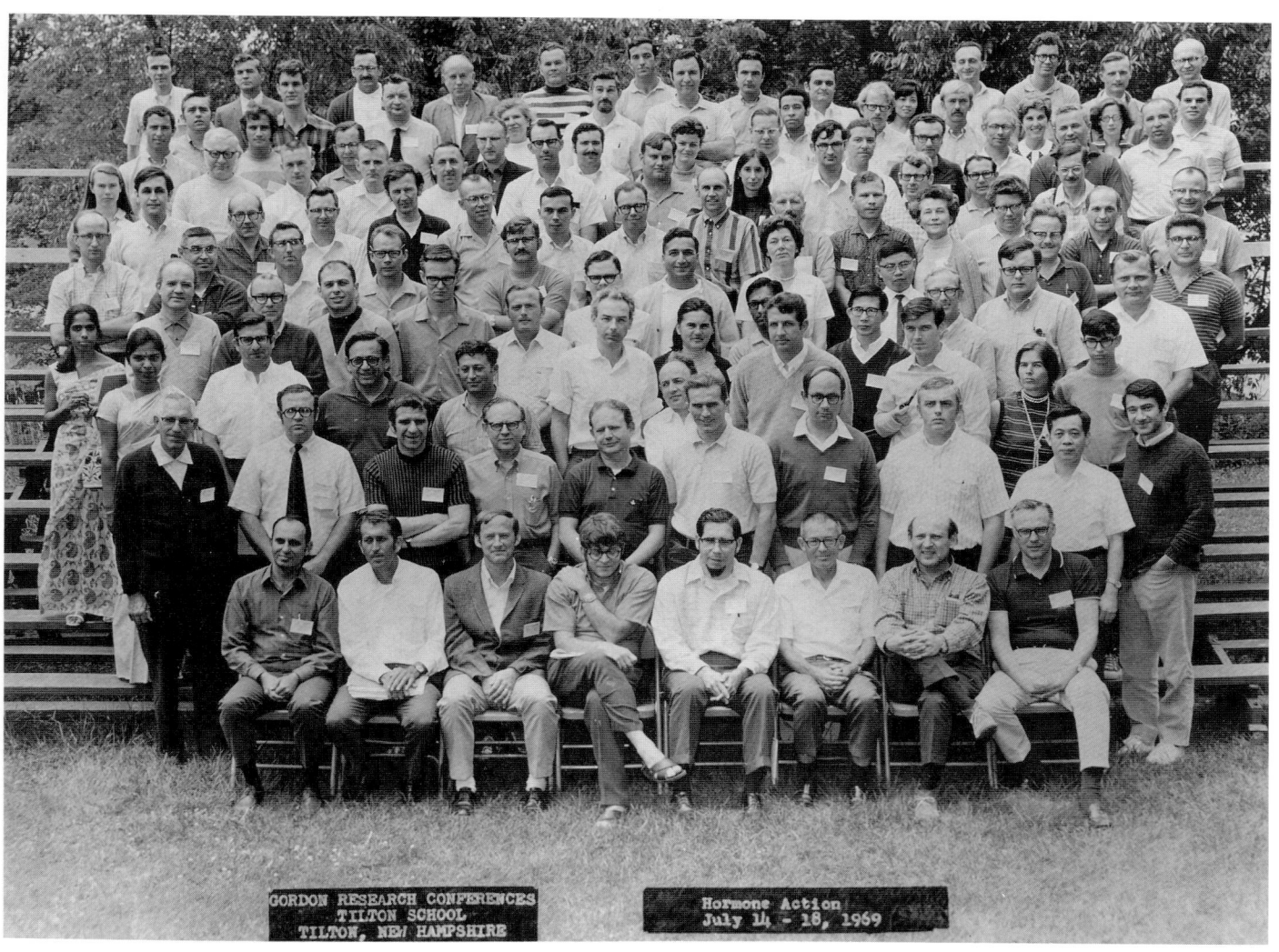

REMEMBRANCE

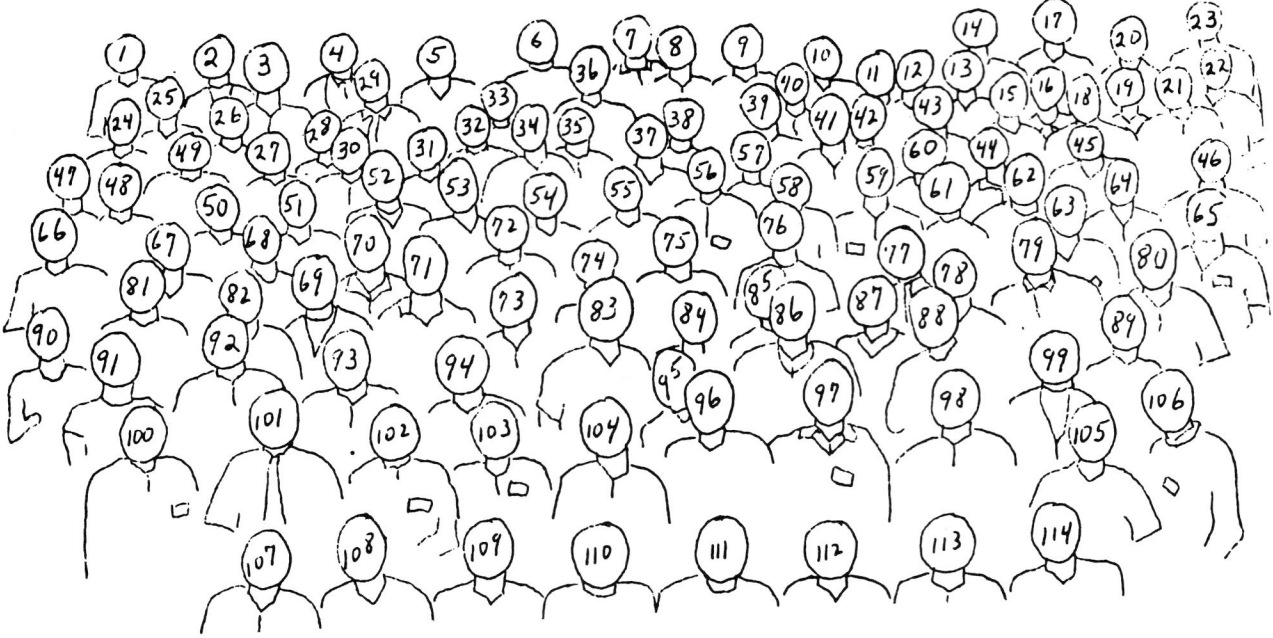

1. J. Castles
2. W. Bencze
3. F. Rolleston
4. G. W. Moersch
5. H. E. Stavely
6. J. J. Ferguson, Jr.
7. E. D. Bransome
8. J. Kowal
9. R. P. Cox
10. F. T. Kenney
11. J. G. Kunkel
12. S. S. Yang
13. R. Klevecz
14. Peter Lengyel
15. G. R. Wyatt
16. I. Bonner
17. J. Warner
18. H. L. Segal
19. Kathleen Birchall
20. E. Brad Thompson
21. Irving Fritz
22. Martin Rodbell
23. J. D. Wilson
24. L. S. Jefferson
25. J. H. Clark
26. Russell Pemberton
27. Kenneth L. Barker
28. George Melnykovych
29. James Tait
30. David Greenman
31. Thomas Mowles
32. Jacques Hanoune
33. Sylvia Tait
34. Reagan H. Bradford
35. David N. Lisi
36. Carl Monder
37. D. Lockwood
38. Jo Milner
39. John A. Franz
40. Ed Peets
41. Angelo Notides
42. G. F. Lata
43. G. Brawerman
44. F. Rosen
45. Dwain Hagerman
46. John C. Babcock
47. Sarah C. R. Elgin
48. George E. Swaneck
49. James C. Warren
50. Claudio Pellegrino
51. Darold Holten
52. T. A. Langan
53. William E. Groves
54. James Rillema
55. Ken Holden
56. Russel J. Kraay
57. Joan Tuttle
58. Jay S. Roth
59. Kenneth Perry
60. Lynn Crook
61. Helen Tepperman
62. Patricia Johnson
63. A. O. Pogo
64. Edgar Henshaw
65. Philip Feigelson
66. Jack Gorski
67. M. S. Glitzer
68. John N. Fain
69. H. M. Goodman
70. George R. Shepherd
71. C. Wayne Bardin
72. C. N. Brewer
73. William L. McGuire
74. Anthony D. Means
75. Richard S. Rivlin
76. Willa Brunkhorst
77. Kai-Lin Lee
78. Fred G. Sherman
79. Jerry R. Reel
80. P. K. Siiteri
81. Hermann Nicmeyer
82. Jack Kostyo
83. Lutz Birnbaumer
84. Genevieve S. Incefy
85. A. H. Reddi
86. Jurgen Drews
87. Fang, Sen-Maw
88. Giovanni A. Puca
89. Eric Feigelson
90. G. Shyamala Harris
91. Leelavati Hurthy
92. Asher Korner
93. Leon L. Miller
94. Joseph Ilan
95. Theodor Braun
96. Hans Peter Bar
97. Alan M. White
98. Bert W. O'Malley
99. Muriel Feigelson
100. Leo T. Samuels
101. Terrell H. Hamilton
102. Ira G. Wool
103. Jay Tepperman
104. Howard M. Katzen
105. Shutsung Liao
106. Etienne Baulieu
107. J. R. Tata
108. Richard G. Cutler
109. W. D. Wicks
110. Gordon Tomkins
111. James R. Florini
112. James Bonner
113. Oscar Hechter
114. Elwood Jensen

Reprinted Copy of 1969 Gordon Research Conference on
Hormone Action Program
Conference Title—Effect of Hormones on RNA and Protein Synthesis

Monday, July 14

James Bonner, "Chemistry of Gene Control"
Gordon M. Tomkins, "Hormonal Regulation of Specific Gene Expression in Mammalian Cells"
Frank T. Kenney, "Hormonal Regulation of Enzyme Synthesis in the Liver"
Wesley D. ('Pete') Wicks, "Role of Cyclic AMP in Regulation of Enzyme Synthesis"
H. P. Bar, "Molecular Aspects of Hormone Action on Membrane-Bound Adenyl Cyclase"

Tuesday, July 15

Elwood V. Jensen, "Estrogen-Receptor Interaction in Target Tissues"
Gerald C. Mueller, "Studies on the Role of Estrogen Receptors in Hormone Response"
Terrell A. Hamilton, "Early Estrogen Action: The Role of Histones and Non-Histone Proteins in the Control of Chromatin Template Activity"
Jack Gorski, "The Effect of Estrogen on the Synthesis of Specific Proteins and RNAs"

Wednesday, July 16

Jean D. Wilson, "The Intranuclear Binding of Testosterone on Rat Prostate"
Shutsung Liao, "Androphilic Proteins and the Mode of Action of Androgens on RNA Synthesis"
James R. Florini, "Effects of Testosterone on RNA Synthesis in Muscle"
Ira G. Wool, "Insulin and the Regulation of Protein Biosynthesis"
Howard M. Katzen, "Insulin in the Regulation of the Soluble and Subcellular Bound Multiple Hexokinases"

Thursday, July 17

Asher Korner, "Growth Hormone and Translational Control of Protein Synthesis"
Jack Kostyo, "Early Effects of Growth Hormone on Protein Metabolism in Muscle"
Jamshed R. Tata, "Coordinated Changes in Cellular Structure and Synthetic Activity during Hormone Action"
Oscar Hechter, "Reflections on the Action of Steroid and Non-Steroid Hormones"

Friday, July 18

Jurgen Drews, "Selective Inhibition by Prednisolone of rRNA Synthesis in Thymus Cells"
Abraham M. White, "The Inhibition of Protein Synthesis in Muscle by Glucocorticoids and Its Reversal by Anabolic Steroids"

The fixed fee for conference participants was $130; resident guests were charged $65 for the week for room and board.

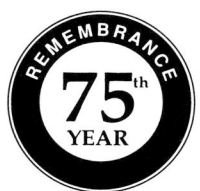

History of the Gordon Conference on Hormone Action

It all started back in '69
In Tilton School in Tilton
When Jim Florini and a couple of guys
Checked into the Cruickshank Hilton

They formed the Hormone Action Club
And agreed to meet each year
To discuss in depth their latest results
And consume large volumes of beer

Some things haven't changed

In '69 we didn't know much
But even then it seemed clear
That chickens were the system of choice
The S.P.C.A. shouldn't hear

Estrogen increased RNA
Gorski knew from the start
But data on this were tough to get
Mother Nature had no heart

At Colby next year with Hechter as chair
There were membranes and cAMP
Phosphorylation the key to it all
But substrates?—Oh, just wait and see

Some things haven't changed

Jay Tepperman chaired it in '71
The meeting reflected his taste
Steroids, sperm, the developing breast
Quite a varied diet we faced

In '73 we came to this place
And learned far too much about bugs
The chair, Jerry Wyatt, had an interest in them
Thank God, his field wasn't slugs

As hormone receptors grew in stature
We measured them quite a lot
George Scatchard became a household term
Though his paper contains no such plot

Along came O'Malley and Schrader, of course
Back then Bert was his preceptor
They lighted the screen in an awesome way
With a funny cigar-shaped receptor

We learned that steroids were found in the brain
Their role was fairly complex
If rat embryos saw the wrong ones first
They wouldn't be sure of their sex

There was Elwood Jensen in '75
With receptors that moved to and fro
They were 8S or 4S or some other size
When he changed salt from high to low

Up jumped Jim Clark with his soft southern drawl
He had different ideas from these
Receptors are nuclear, he maintained
They don't move about as they please

One year when things were kind of slow
We thought we'd move to the sun
Santa Barbara meeting in wintertime
Sounded like lots of fun

So, we tore ourselves away from our labs
My—what disappointment we feigned
We packed our rackets and summer gear
When we got there it rained and it rained

The Hotel Miramar was our site
A railroad ran right through it
At 2 o'clock every single night
When the train came by, you knew it

The food was atrocious, you couldn't believe
What they could do to meat
After two days of meals, there were vacant chairs
Those who could, went out to eat

But the science was tip-top as ever
And the parties were pretty cool
At the oddest times, those dark rainy nights
We fished people out of the pool

Remember the night the power went out
We lit candles and kept on talking
'til the firechief arrived and with no sense of humor
Threw us out amidst plenty of squawking

Received May 2, 1991.
"Remembrance," articles discuss people and events as remembered by the author. The opinion(s) expressed are solely those of the writer and do not reflect the view of the Journal or The Endocrine Society.

REMEMBRANCE

After two year's time we could no longer bear
the site of that food on the plate
So we took a vote—the results were clear cut
Go back East where the lobsters were great

In Plymouth, we suffered through blistering heat
In a dorm with a lovely pool table
Sleeping was out of the question that year
With the heat and the noise who was able?

Michael Conn entertained us with publishing jokes
of reviewers with an acid pen
He made fun of the process and rightfully so
Who'd have thought he'd be editor then

In '81 we had no conference
The chairs forgot to arrange one
I'll bet they took a lot of heat
Before that summer was done

By '82 we'd come 'round to thinking
Peptide hormones were hot
Kinase C with its strange phospholipids
Made us learn structures, like it or not

That was also the year they told us
A message for insulin existed
It was peptide—no! lipid—no! sugar or what
No shortage of theories persisted

By '83 we were growing big rats
By putting in growth hormone genes
Ron Evans forgot to bring his slides
His memory had failed him it seems

The threat of all this to the country was clear
Researchers were playing God
The next thing you know, they'll be patenting rats
Jerry Falwell pronounced it a fraud

Committment of genes and the hormone response
Were topics in '84
If you're having feeling of déjà vu
It's because we've discussed this before

In '85 Marc Lipman came through
With a speaker on insect mating
The intimate sex life of bugs in detail
The talk got a triple "X" rating

In '86, we started the week
With a dinner of scallops and more
Then a strange thing happened at the end of each talk
Half the audience raced for the door.

Because Daryl Granner was moving his lab
Stan Korenmann cochaired that year
Daryl made the program and raised all the cash
And Korenman sponsored the beer

Ira Herskowitz came to us the next year
He told us of love-making yeasts
They need factors and kinase and God knows what else
They're very fastidious beasts

Last year, development caught our attention
We suddenly started to see
That hormones were playing a major role
In deciding what we would be

And, speaking of growth and development, friends
There are plenty of people in town
Who think it's arrested in many of us
Or at least, it's been slowed way down

I refer, of course, to Thursday, last year
When some of you went on a spree
Staggering throught the campus streets
You sang songs 'til a quarter past three

For 20 years this conference was good
In spite of some abberations
We've had first rate speakers in lots of fields
And they've come from several nations

This year, we've heard peptides and kinases, too
And calcium's still to come
We've learned that a protein for IGF II
Builds a matrix that looks like gum

It seems that steroids enhance transcription
Or else they turn it off
They bind to the DNA structure
At a place that looks like a trough

It looks like the site is hidden from view
But receptor still finds its home
Thanks to proteins in clusters and groups
That form a nucleosome

I've learned a lot from the steroid people
Some of those techniques are neat
But one thing that bothers me still today
Is that footprints don't look much like feet

Someone has mentioned there's fashion in science
That certainly seems to be true
At first, we were flooded with northern blots
Now its gel shifts and zinc fingers too

Now that the time is drawing near
To pass on the conference to others
Some words of advice are in order, I think
From us veterans to our soul brothers

REMEMBRANCE

Although we've discussed all the problems I guess
Over the last 20 years
There are still some fantastic things out there
To excite our eyes and our ears

Your job will be really quite simple
Invite those people who best
Keep their listeners spellbound for hours
And they will do all the rest

Of course, the money to pay for them
Is limited quite severely
You pray that they'll buy Apex tickets
So it won't hit your budget too dearly.

There's one other thing that's important to say
Denis Reisch is a valuable friend
He oils the conference machinery for you
From Sunday right through to the end

In conclusion, I guess we should tell you
What great fun this year has been
But it's nice to have Carter and Gordon out there
Since we'd rather not do this again.

                          Frances Finn
                    Protein Research Laboratory

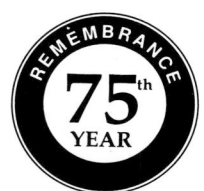

Memoir—The Beginning of Oral Contraceptives

As we filed into the conference room at the Searle Laboratories in Skokie, Illinois, none of us realized then that we were participating in an historical occasion, or that we were starting a revolution. The meeting that followed had been called by I. C. Winter, Medical Director of Searle, later Vice President. Winter, a physician who also held a doctorate in pharmacology, was temporary Director of Biological Research while the company searched for a senior biologist, a position later filled by Victor A. Drill. During the meeting, Winter, or I. C. as he was known, explained that he had just returned from a meeting where, in discussion with various physicians, he had identified a medical need for an orally effective progestational agent to be used therapeutically for habitual abortion, endometriosis, dysmenorrhea, and control of irregular menstrual cycles; he suggested that we go find one.

Searle was a propitious place for such an effort—the research division was already committed to a steroid program. It was the summer of 1952. The structure of cortisone had recently been defined by Kendall and Hench had shown its therapeutic potential in arthritis; Reichstein, the Taits, and others were surveying the adrenal effluent for other active compounds; the gonadal steroids had been defined structurally during the 1930s, but the second World War had prevented extensive therapeutic exploitation of these agents. However, estrogens, both natural steroids and synthetic steroid analogs and testosterone were used for various deficiency states and injectable progesterone was employed in an effort to salvage pregnancies in women who miscarried regularly. Pharmaceutical scientists were actively searching for corticoids, for new estrogens, particularly nonsteroidal agents related to stilbestrol, and anabolic agents that had the metabolic effects of testosterone, but lacked its masculinizing effects. Searle was one of the more aggressive companies in this regard, building up to a steroid group of some 40 synthetic organic chemists, supported by a series of endocrinologists that started with Francis J. Saunders and me. Initially, Saunders and I tried to cover all bases, but we were soon joined by Lee G. Hershberger and Charles M. Kagawa from R. K. Meyer's lab at Wisconsin and Richard L. Elton, a student of M. X. Zarrow from Purdue. The final organization had Saunders working primarily on the androgens, Hershberger on glucocorticoids, Kagawa on mineralocorticoids, Elton on progestagens, and me on estrogens and their antagonists. Significant input to the program was also provided by Gregory Pincus of the Worcester Foundation who functioned as a consultant.

As a result of this burgeoning steroid program, Searle Research was ready when Frank Colton synthesized norethynodrel in 1952. The year before Carl Djerassi of Syntex had synthesized norethindrone, but at the time Syntex was a small Mexican chemical company lacking in biological or medical departments, and was not prepared rapidly to exploit newly prepared compounds. Norethynodrel and a range of other structural relatives of 19-nortestosterone were studied in the Skokie Laboratories and were submitted to the Worcester Foundation for evaluation. Work carried out at Worcester was summarized by Pincus and associates in 1956, while Searle work was presented by Drill and Riegel at the Laurentian Hormone Conference in 1957.

By the mid-1950s ideas about the therapeutic use of progestagens had expanded and their potential as contraceptives was recognized. Clinical evaluation of norethynodrel as a contraceptive was actively pursued by John Rock in Boston and by Celso-Ramon Garcia and Edris Rice-Wray in Puerto Rico, while Edward T. Tyler was evaluating norethindrone in Los Angeles. It soon became apparent that progestagens alone were not satisfactory as contraceptives and that an estrogen was also needed to control abnormal uterine bleeding. The incorporation of estrogens in oral contraceptive formulations was the result of clinical observations and bioassays carried out in my laboratory. This was, of course, before the identification of receptors, a decade later, or the development of RIA techniques: quantification was based on uterine growth or vaginal cornification in rodents, but these assays were superior to chemical techniques available at the time.

Understanding the need for estrogen is itself an interesting story. The early samples of norethynodrel and norethindrone were contaminated with the 3-methyl ether of ethynyl estradiol, now known as mestranol, an intermediate in the synthesis of norethynodrel, which itself was the penultimate intermediate in the synthesis

---

Received March 25, 1991.

"Remembrance," articles discuss people and events as remembered by the author. The opinion(s) expressed are solely those of the writer and do not reflect the view of the Journal or The Endocrine Society.

of norethindrone. As purification of the progestagen proceeded, the incidence of intermenstrual bleeding in women increased leading to the incorporation of fixed amounts of first mestranol and later ethynyl estradiol in the final preparation. It was I. C. Winter who fixed on the contraceptive combination of 0.150 mg mestranol with 9.85 mg norethynodrel, which was marketed by Searle in 1960 as Enovid. Two years later norethindrone at 10 mg with mestranol at 0.06 mg was marketed by Ortho under license by Syntex. This was soon followed by a spate of preparations that combined various progestagens with mestranol or ethynyl estradiol and the race to reduce dose of first the progestagen and later the estrogen began.

In the U.S. over the next decade Syntex released norethindrone/mestranol, Parke Davis, norethindrone acetate and ethynyl estradiol, Searle ethynodiol diacetate and mestranol, Wyeth norgestrel and EE, while Upjohn and Lilly marketed preparations based on acetoxyprogesterone derivatives.

In the 30 years since Enovid was first marketed, the progestagens related to 19-nortestosterone have continued to dominate the oral contraceptive market while those based on progesterone itself have disappeared in the U.S. at least. Norethynodrel, also, has vanished from the oral contraceptive market: as early as the late 1950s and early 1960s it was apparent that the conjugated form, norethindrone, was superior to its $\Delta^{5(10)}$ analog. Newer progestagens such as desogestrel, norgestimate, and gestodene are norgestrel derivatives, basically nortestosterones, but their long-term success remains to be determined. However, that research conference in 1952 led to the first oral contraceptive, which sparked the "sexual revolution" and permitted aspects of the feminist movement as we know it now. It was a good meeting—I'm glad I was there.

Richard A. Edgren
Director
Scientific Affairs
Syntex Laboratories, Inc.

References

1. Pincus G, Chang MC, Zarrow MX, Hafez ESE, Merrill A 1956 Studies of the biological activity of certain 19-nor steroids in female animals. Endocrinology 59:695–707
2. Drill VA, Riegel B 1958 Structural and hormonal activity of some new steroids. Recent Prog Hormone Res 14:29–67

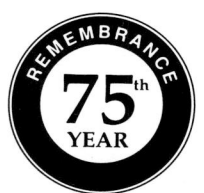

The 1959 West Point Conference on Mechanisms Concerned with Conception: A Landmark Event in Endocrinology

Few among us are privileged to participate in research symposia that have profound and direct influences on both the direction of scientific inquiry and on subsequent industrial developments. The Symposium on Mechanisms Concerned with Conception, held at West Point, NY in July 1959 under the auspices of the Population Council and the Planned Parenthood Federation of America, was such a conference and those of us who attended knew almost immediately that a number of important developments in the endocrine world were about to occur.

The list of 70-odd invited participants in the conference now reads like a Who's Who of Endocrinology and Reproductive Biology. Many are now retired and a number are deceased. Without exception they have made lasting contributions to the field.

Gregory Pincus reported the results of the first large scale clinical trials with orally active ovulation-inhibiting steroids, and it was clear that a contraceptive drug industry was likely to develop. Those of us interested in reproduction in farm animals also realized the potential of these drugs for synchronizing the estrous cycles of cattle and the first successful trials were carried out within the year. M. C. Chang reported the first successful *in vitro* fertilization resulting in birth of live young and the potential for commercial *in vitro* fertilization and embryo transfer in man and the domestic animals became obvious.

However, in the long-term these reports were probably of no greater significance than those concerning the role of the hypothalamus in the neuroendocrine control of the anterior pituitary and ovary. Jack Everett presented convincing evidence for the now generally accepted concepts that eventually led to the isolation of LHRH and other hypothalmic neurohumors. During the discussion, Sir Solly Zuckerman, the General Chairman of the conference, who disagreed with these concepts, seized upon our own results showing that administration of oxytocin to cattle during the early part of the estrous cycle resulted in inhibition of corpus luteum development and a shortened estrous cycle, as proof that the "pituitary portal vessels are an unnecessary speculative adjunct to the proposition that the hypothalamus may be involved". However, even at this early date, we knew that the presence of the uterus was necessary for oxytocin to exert its effects on ovarian function, and with help of others in the audience, were able to use this and other information to defend the concept of hypothalamic production of neurohumors and their transport to the pituitary by the portal vascular system. It is difficult to estimate the impact these discussions may have had on subsequent decisions to support and carry out research on the hypothalamus, but for many of us they were critical.

Despite the oppressive heat and humidity in the old Thayer Hotel, where the meetings were held, the conference was not without its humorous moments. C. R. Austin presented convincing evidence showing that sperm capacitation is associated with detachment of the acrosome. M. C. Chang arose during the ensuing discussion to report that he had "decapacitated" rabbit sperm by suspending them in bull seminal plasma. He (Chang) then asked Austin, "Do you suppose that I put the acrosomes back on these rabbit sperm when I resuspended them in bull seminal plasma?!"

The proceedings of the conference [Mechanisms Concerned with Conception, the MacMillan Co., New York, 1963, C. G. Hartman (ed)] were long delayed in publication and, for the most part, failed to highlight the most important developments of the conference, particularly those that were destined to have practical applications leading to the establishment of new industries. Nonetheless, the proceedings served as a valuable reference for many years and a particularly valuable "Inventory of Unanswered Questions" was included in the appendix. Even today this section is worth reading because many of these questions remain unanswered.

William Hansel
Gordon D. Cain
Professor of Animal Physiology
Louisiana State University

Received May 17, 1991.

"Remembrance," articles discuss people and events as remembered by the author. The opinion(s) expressed are solely those of the writer and do not reflect the view of the Journal or The Endocrine Society.

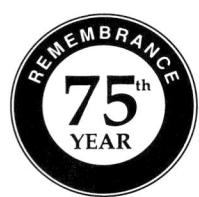

The Backstage Story of the Discovery of LHRH

During my postdoctoral years (1956–1961) spent first at Yale University and then at Tulane University, I was fortunate to become acquainted with many talented endocrinologists. At that time, my major interest was the role of vasopressin in stimulating ACTH secretion. Vasopressin was then one of the strongest candidates for CRF, as advocated by Don McCann. Roger Guillemin and Andrew Schally claimed the existence of separate CRF-α and CRF-β molecules. At Tulane University I worked with Joseph Dingman in the Department of Medicine where I tried to establish a method for separating vasopressin from human plasma using glass fiber paper chromatography. In 1960, on the way home from Miami after attending the Annual Endocrinology Meeting, I happened to board the plane with Schally. He showed a considerable interest in the chromatographic method on which I was working. We talked enthusiastically about CRF and he emphatically denied the possibility that vasopressin was CRF. During my stay in New Orleans, I visited Guillemin and Schally at Baylor College a couple of times. In contrast to Guillemin, a European professor type, Schally was always working feverishly beside his column. One day when I visited him he was watching the column-electrophoresis with reddened eyes, telling me that he watched the column to purify CRF for 2 days without sleep. I began to feel sympathy with Schally, thinking that some day I could help him.

In the summer of 1961, I returned to Japan. Six months later, I received a letter from Schally asking me to join his new peptide laboratory in New Orleans at the VA Hospital where he had recently moved from Houston. To assure my future security in the USA and accept Schally's invitation, I needed an immigration visa. He urged me to come back to Tulane to work with him as soon as possible, but I had no idea when I would reach the limited quota for Asian immigration. Schally kept me informed in detail of the progress of his research in purifying TRH, GRF, CRF, PIF, LH-, and FSH-releasing hormone. He said he desperately needed a competent physiologist to win the race for the isolation of hypothalamic hypophysiotropic hormones. He offered an equal partnership in which he would be responsible for the chemical purification work, while I would be responsible for all physiological studies including assaying for releasing and inhibiting hormones. I had two very competent graduate students in my physiology laboratory in Sapporo. Although they had not yet completed their Ph.D. work, they were well trained in several skills necessary for endocrine research. So, I asked these students, Akihiro Kuroshima, now Chairman of the Department of Physiology, Asahikawa Medical College, and Yuichi Ishida, now a well known endocrinologist in Sapporo, to go to New Orleans to help Schally until I could join him. Between 1963 and 1965 they worked admirably to optimize the bioassays for screening fractions for bioactivity during purification. In 1965, I had still not obtained an immigration visa. A friendly American Consul in Sapporo suggested to me that I obtain support for my joining Tulane/VA's research team from the Department of Defense so that the State Department could issue a special permit for me to go and work in New Orleans before acquiring my immigration visa. Schally immediately followed the Consul's advice. He told me later that the Pentagon soon called him asking about the importance of the LHRH research he needed me for the defense of America. He made a very realistic if hyperbolic proposal describing the possible application of an LHRH antagonist in the defense program. I received a letter from the State Department, requesting my immediate departure from Japan to join Schally's team. In March 1965, I came back to Tulane to join the race for the research in hypophysiotropic hormones.

The bioassays used for the purification of the hypophysiotropic hormones were based on measuring changes in blood levels of pituitary hormones or change in the hormone content of the pituitary after injection of a test sample. The pituitary hormones in blood or tissue were determined by another bioassay. Therefore, the bioassay for hypophysiotropic hormones required two bioassays in series, both extremely tedious, time consuming, expensive, and not very accurate. In the late 1960s, reports of a RIA for pituitary hormones began to appear, but most were of the method for nonrat hormones. As soon as a RIA method for ovine PRL was reported by Li and Arai in Endocrinology, I contacted them in Denver and obtained their permission to learn the technique there. I flew to Denver. The method was straightforward, but they used gel electrophoresis for purifying the labeled

---

Received April 9, 1991.

"Remembrance" articles discuss people and events as remembered by the author. The opinion(s) expressed are solely those of the writer and do not reflect the view of the Journal or The Endocrine Society.

PRL. Since gel filtration on Sephadex was routine at Schally's lab, I used this method for purifying the tracer. It worked well. Around this time, Gordon Niswender, then at the University of Michigan, generated his famous rabbit antiovine LH, no. 15, which cross-reacted with LH from all mammalian species, including rat LH. He was very generous, cooperative, and helpful when I asked him to supply us with his no. 15 LH antiserum. Without his help and his no. 15 antiserum, the screening of LHRH could not have proceeded swiftly, and purification of LHRH would have been considerably delayed. The critical bioassay step was also nearly perfect. The method developed at McCann's laboratory empolying ovariectomized, estradiol- and progesterone-treated rats, showed satisfactory sensitivity and accuracy in terms of LH release induced by crude hypothalamic extracts as well as purified LHRH preparation. The requirement for the assay for hypophysiotropic hormone was 1) sensitivity, 2) specificity, 3) reproducibility, 4) accuracy, 5) practicality. Our routine LHRH assay system completely fulfilled these requirements.

In the 60s, Schally had succeeded in isolating about 250 μg LHRH from 160,000 porcine hypothalami. A Japanese chemist Yoshihiko Baba and I tried to characterize its structure. In contrast to advanced facility for purification at Schally's laboratory, the instruments for analytical chemistry were second rate. Baba struggled with a shakey amino acid analyzer patiently, and finally managed to reveal the presence of the nine amino acids in LHRH molecule. Various chemical and enzymatic treatments of purified LHRH were performed to examine the effects on the biological activity. I returned the bioassay result to Baba in as short a time as was possible, so that Baba could design the next step of the experiment. The information obtained from these studies helped us to understand some physiochemical characteristics and possible amino acid pairs in the molecule.

Pyroglutamyl peptidase prepared by Russell Doolittle inactivated LHRH, suggesting the presence of pGlu at the N-terminus, that was also reported by Guillemin's group. But, Doolittle's enzyme was found to split LHRH into more than two fragments, indicating that the enzyme was not pure. After another Japanese chemist Hisayuki Matsuo joined us, I asked Doolittle for the highly purified enzyme preparation. He promised to bring it with him when he came to New Orleans to attend a meeting. He wanted us to use a sufficient amount of his enzyme to inactivate LHRH, and he indeed brought us the enzyme in an amount more than enough. But we still worried about its purity. We wanted to have a decisive answer as whether LHRH indeed had pGlu at the N-terminus. So, in order to avoid possible cleavage of the peptide by another enzyme contaminants in Doolittle's preparation, we wanted to use a minimum amount of the enzyme preparation. He could not understand why we insisted on using a smaller amount than he recommended. He wanted us to demonstrate a splendid activity of his enzyme in destroying LHRH activity. While traveling in the car returning him to the airport he scolded us to urge us to use a larger amount of enzyme. But finally he seemed to understand our view. His highly purified enzyme inactivated LHRH at a very small concentration.

At this time, HPLC had not been developed and the conventional method for structural analysis of blocked peptides included enzymatic degradation, purification, and isolation of the resulting fragments, followed by Edman degradation, required much larger amount of the peptide. So, 250 μg of the peptide were absolutely not enough. When a certain sequence was predicted, it must be verified by synthesis. No peptide synthesizer was available in our lab. I believed that Schally intended to ask Abbott to synthesize the peptide for us. He considered the peptide synthesis could be done by any person. But Baba and I agreed that the predicted sequence must be confirmed by synthesis ourselves. A manual peptide synthesizer was not so expensive, and Baba had confidence he could synthesize the peptide by himself. Schally did not show much interest in purchasing the synthesizer, but we insisted on its necessity. I consulted with C. G. Huggins, Professor of Biochemistry at Tulane University about the instruments. He agreed with us and provided me with information on a peptide synthesizer. The instrument was available from Daikin Co., Osaka, Japan. I ordered it immediately. The instrument arrived in late 1970.

Schally asked me if there were any extremely competent Japanese chemists who could solve the problem of using 250 μg material on hand. I wrote a letter to my friend Keizo Asami, Professor of Keio University School of Medicine, asking if he knew any such chemist. I knew Asami had a marvelous network of information on human resources. He discussed with his fellow professor Seiichi Inayama, Director of Institute of Pharmaceutical Chemistry of Keio. Inayama soon recommended to me a chemist and sent me his CV. The chemist seemed to be competent, but not extraordinarily, judging from the CV. I explained Inayama the problem which we had to solve. Inayama presented my request to the Committee of Professors at Tokyo University Faculty of Pharmaceutical Chemistry. I was informed that it would be impossible to characterize the structure of LHRH structure using such a small amount with currently available analytical methods. Inayama continued his effort to find a solution. When he read a report of a new method for identifying the C-terminus of a peptide using a selective ^{3}H-labeling, he thought the method which required a very small amount of peptide could be used for determining the structure of LHRH. The method was developed by Hisayuki Matsuo, Protein Institute, Osaka. Inayama wrote to me that Matsuo was the chemist whom we were looking for. He urged me to persuade Matsuo to join Schally's team. I did write many letters to Matsuo. Although he initially did not show much interest in my invitation, he gradually inclined to think about testing his untested method for a practical problem: the determination of LHRH structure using a small amount of material.

Matsuo and his wife arrived in New Orleans on New Year's Eve 1970. He seemed shocked by the outdated analytical instruments in our laboratory, but surprised and very impressed by Schally's bluntness and such trust that he made his whole stock of purified LHRH available to Matsuo. The second shock came soon to all of us. Neither the VA or Tulane University had the license needed to order 0.5 Ci tritiated water, the minimum ordering amount. The officials of the VA Hospital told me that it would take a long time, several months to a year, to obtain the license. Matsuo could not use his method for selective tritium labeling unless he had tritiated water. I was desparate, and sought help from LSU which I hoped might have an institutional license for purchasing 0.5 Ci tritiated water. I met Ernest A. Daigneault, Professor of Pharmacology, who was in charge of radioisotopes at LSU Medical School. The problem was solved. He was very helpful and cooperative. He not only agreed to purchase the radioisotope at LSU, but also permitted Matsuo to perform his initial experiment at his laboratory under LSU license. I was so grateful to him. Now Matsuo did not have to return to Japan without doing any experiments!

Matsuo confirmed that his method worked satisfactorily for determining the C-terminus using only a few micrograms of lysine vasopressin as a model peptide, which also has amidated C-terminus as would be the case for LHRH. Matsuo made a brave gamble. Matsuo's gamble was to determine N- and C-terminal amino acids of fragments generated by digestion of Schally's purified LHRH by chymotrypsin or thermolysin without further purification. Baba determined N-terminal amino acids using microscale Edman degradation, and Matsuo determined C-terminal amino acid using selective tritium labeling. The number of N-terminal amino acids was supposed to be the same as that of C-terminal amino acids, but it was not. The experiment went wrong or we overlooked an amino acid. Matsuo found that Trp which is destroyed by ordinary acid hydrolysis was overlooked. LHRH had not 9, but 10 amino acids. It was very important information. Trp had also been overlooked by Guillemin's team. From a jigsaw game-like trial using N- and C-terminal amino acids of mixed enzyme-digested fragments followed by a few steps of Edman degradation, the two most likely candidates for LHRH structure were postulated. Since Baba went to a meeting in California with Schally, Matsuo started synthesizing the first candidate peptide using the new peptide synthesizer which arrived from Japan. As soon as he gave me the synthetic material, I injected the material into the assay rats. Blood was collected for LH assays by RIA using Niswender's antiserum.

Sunday, April 25, 1971 was a beautiful day. When I left my home, I told my wife that today might become a memorable day in the history of neuroendocrinology and asked her to prepare for a celebration if I found the LH-releasing activity in the synthetic material prepared by Matsuo. Strangely, the hubcap of my car fell off twice during driving to work. It had never happened before. Although I didn't pay attention to omens, it was not a pleasant experience on such an important day.

The second floor of the lab was quiet and empty. I removed test tubes from the refrigerator and centrifuged. I sat in front of the auto-γ-counter and watched the register. Suddenly, the counting started falling, indicating a tremendous release of LH. I knew first in the world the structure and activity of LHRH. It was 9:00 a.m. I called Matsuo. His wife told me that he was still sleeping. He started synthesizing the second candidate for LHRH and came home at 3:00 a.m. I told her to wake him up, he wouldn't mind being awakened. He came to the phone and greeted me with a sleepy voice. I told him that the synthetic material showed a tremendous LH-releasing activity. His voice suddenly changed as if he misunderstood my message. He promised to come to the lab immediately. I also called Baba. He was out. Then I went downstairs to see Schally. He used to work at his office in the morning of every Sunday. I said quietly "Andrew, we finally got it. Congratulations." We shook hands. I saw a smile started spreading on Schally's face. I called my wife to share my excitement with her. In the evening, Schally and his wife, Baba, Matsuo and his wife, and my wife and I celebrated altogether for the discovery of LHRH at a champagne and steak dinner at a small dining room in my home at Chelsea Drive.

Akira Arimura
US-Japan Biomedical Laboratory
Tulane University Herbert Center

Acknowledgment

The author is grateful to Dr. Brenda Shivers for her valuable advice and excellent editorial assistance in preparing this manuscript.

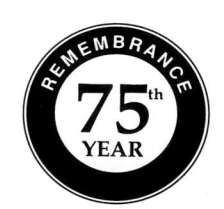

Why I was Told not to Study Inhibin and What I did about it

We entered the inhibin field accidentally. We were trying to account for our failure to inhibit serum FSH in the ovariectomized rat with estradiol plus progesterone. We were also puzzled by what accounted for the secondary FSH surge which follows the preovulatory gonadotropin surges in the rodent. It had been shown by others that once the primary surges occurred, the prolonged rise in serum FSH lasting to estrus was not dependent on further GnRH action. We wondered if the preovulatory LH surge turned off secretion from the ovary of an FSH-suppressing substance simultaneously with causing resumption of meiosis and ovulation (1, 2).

These observations suggested that another feedback hormone from the ovary might specifically be responsible for FSH negative feedback. But that sounded like the elusive nonsteroidal substance "inhibin" that scientists working with testicular feedback had been searching for since the early 1920s (3). Because of the failure to purify such a substance after so many years, the field was seen as "questionable" by many scientists.

In the mid 1970s the late Cornelia (Nina) Channing, of the Department of Physiology, University of Maryland School of Medicine, was engaged in a search for an ovarian "oocyte meiosis inhibitor" (OMI). It had been known for some time that mammalian oocytes explanted within their surrounding follicles did not exhibit germinal vesicle breakdown (GVB) or resumption of meiosis. However, if the oocytes within cumulus were explanted after removal from their surrounding follicles, they resumed meiosis quickly. These observations led some reproductive scientists, including Channing, to postulate that endogenous follicular fluid contained an OMI which was suppressed by the preovulatory LH surge, allowing the rapid GVB and meiosis resumption seen on the afternoon of proestrus in the rat.

Channing and colleagues (4) had shown that porcine follicular fluid (pFF) contained a peptide which could at least partly suppress or delay GVB in explanted follicles. It occurred to me that the same OMI could be our hypothetical FSH-suppressing substance, since both activities were postulated to be reduced by the natural LH

Received June 7, 1991.

"Remembrance" articles discuss people and events as remembered by the author. The opinoion(s) expressed are solely those of the writer and do not reflect the view of the Journal or The Endocrine Society.

surge. I called Nina and she agreed to send me some charcoal extracted pFF to test on the secondary FSH surge in the female rat. We injected it after the primary gonadotropin surges were complete, and collected blood at 0400 h of estrus, when the secondary FSH surge was maximum. To our great satisfaction, pFF caused a major fall in serum FSH, which was dose dependent! We submitted an abstract to the FASEB 1977 meeting, and then sent an expanded paper to PNAS (5). In that paper we suggested naming the substance "folliculostatin," since it suppressed FSH secretion, but the name never caught on outside our own laboratories, and the substance continued to be called "inhibin."

In the meantime DeJong and Sharpe (6) had shown that bovine FF could suppress serum FSH selectively in castrated male rats, scooping us in the demonstration that FF was a better source of inhibin than was testicular extract.

After the FASEB meeting in early 1977, where I presented the paper, I received several phone calls from good friends in endocrinology, and I suppose that Nina did also, counseling me "not to get into the inhibin field." The rationale was that it seemed strange that people had searched for so long to no avail, and that while some laboratories claimed to have a partially purified inhibin other laboratories could not confirm it. Thus, many scientists had concluded it did not exist. In retrospect, the probable reasons for the lag in the field were several: testicular extract does not contain as high a concentration of inhibin as FF; the *in vivo* bioassays were never standardized and were insensitive; the male bioassay recipient is not as sensitive to inhibin as the female (2).

Nina and I went on to show that OMI and inhibin were not the same molecule, since the FSH-suppressing activity was in the greater than 10,000 mol wt fraction, whereas OMI was in the greater than 2,000 mol wt fraction (7). As it turned out, conventional biochemical protein isolation techniques never yielded isolation of inhibin, but the techniques of molecular biology were successful in identifying the two subunits of inhibin in four laboratories simultaneously (8–11). Unfortunately, Nina died just before the existence of the inhibin molecule was confirmed. The issue of what substance in pFF is OMI is still controversial (12).

Why did I persist in looking for ovarian inhibin in the face of so many friendly warnings from respected colleagues and in the light of a 50-year history of unresolved research on testicular inhibin? For two reasons, I think. Had I been more junior in my career in the mid-70s I might have abandoned the search for fear of adding myself to the long list of investigators who had failed to confirm the existence of inhibin. As it was, I assumed that I could survive the possible failure if it occurred. Additionally, however, our physiological analysis of ovarian/pituitary relationships demanded another feedback hormone from the ovary! Something had to account for the relative nonsuppressibility of serum FSH after ovariectomy, and for the prolonged postsurge FSH rise in rats and hamsters. And I was stubborn enough to take the chance that follicular fluid might contain the nonsteroidal hormone. Consequently, it was a real high to show, with Kelly Mayo's laboratory, that messenger RNA for inhibin subunits declined on the afternoon of proestrus (13). Finally, using a RIA for the α-inhibin subunit, it has been possible to demonstrate that serum inhibin drops on the afternoon of proestrus, just as we had predicted (14)!

Neena B. Schwartz
Department of Neurobiology/Physiology
Northwestern University

References

1. Schwartz N, Talley W 1978 Effects of exogenous LH or FSH on endogenous FSH, progesterone and estradiol secretion. Biol Reprod 18:820–828
2. Grady R, Charlesworth MC, Schwartz NB 1982 Characterization of the FSH-suppressing activity in follicular fluid. In: Greep RO (ed) Recent Progress Hormone Research. Academic Press, New York, vol 38:409–456
3. DeJong FH 1988 Inhibin. Physiol Rev 68:555–607
4. Tsafriri A, Pomerantz SH, Channing CP 1976 Inhibition of oocyte maturation by porcine follicular fluid: partial characterization of the inhibitor. Biol Reprod 14:511–516
5. Schwartz NB, Channing CP 1977 Evidence for ovarian "inhibin" suppression of the secondary rise in serum follicle stimulating hormone levels in proestrous rats by injection of porcine follicular fluid. Proc Natl Acad Sci USA 74:5721–5724
6. DeJong FH, Sharpe RM 1976 Evidence for inhibin-like activity in bovine follicular fluid. Nature 263:71–72
7. Lorenzen JR, Channing CP, Schwartz NB 1978 Partial characterization of FSH-suppressing activity (folliculostatin) in porcine follicular fluid using the metestrous rat as an in vivo model. Biol Reprod 19:635–640
8. Robertson DM, Foulds LM, Lerersha L, Morgan FJ, Hearn MTW, Burger HG, Wetenhall REH, deKretser DM 1985 Isolation of inhibin from bovine follicular fluid. Biochem Biophys Res Commun 126:220–226
9. Miyamoto K, Hasegawa Y, Fukuda M, Nomura M, Igarashi M, Kangawa K, Matsuo H 1985 Isolation of porcine follicular fluid inhibin of 32K daltons. Biochem Biophys Res Commun 129:396–403
10. Rivier J, Spiess J, McClintock R, Vaughan J, Vale W 1985 Purification and partial characterization of inhibin from porcine follicular fluid. Biochem Biophys Res Commun 133:120–127
11. Ling N, Ying S-Y, Ueno N, Esch F, Denoroy L, Guillemin R 1985 Isolation and partial characterization of a Mr 32,000 protein with inhibin activity from porcine follicular fluid. Proc Natl Acad Sci USA 82:7217–7221
12. Tsafriri A 1988 Local nonsteroidal regulators of ovarian function. In: Knobil E, Neill JD (eds) The Physiology of Reproduction. Raven Press, New York, pp 527–565
13. Woodruff TK, D'Agostino JB, Schwartz NB, Mayo KE 1988 Dynamic changes in inhibin mRNAs in rat ovarian follicles during the reproductive cycle. Science 239:1296–1299
14. Ackland JF, D'Agostino JB, Ringstrom SJ, Hostetler JP, Mann BG, Schwartz NB 1990 Circulating radioimmunoassayable inhibin during periods of transient FSH rise: secondary surge and unilateral ovariectomy. Biol Reprod 43:347–352

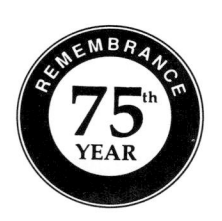

Remembrance of H. W. Magoun's Contributions to the Development of Neuroendocrinology

The recent death in March 1991, of one of this century's foremost neuroscientists, Dr. H. W. Magoun (Fig. 1), recalls that his seminal research on the structure and function of the hypothalamus in the 1930s laid a cornerstone for the development of neuroendocrinology. In Ranson's Institute of Neurology at Northwestern University Medical School in Chicago Magoun and his colleagues demonstrated that specific areas of the hypothalamus exert controls not only over feeding, drinking, body temperature, and sleep but also over certain pituitary functions and animal behavior related to reproduction and water metabolism.

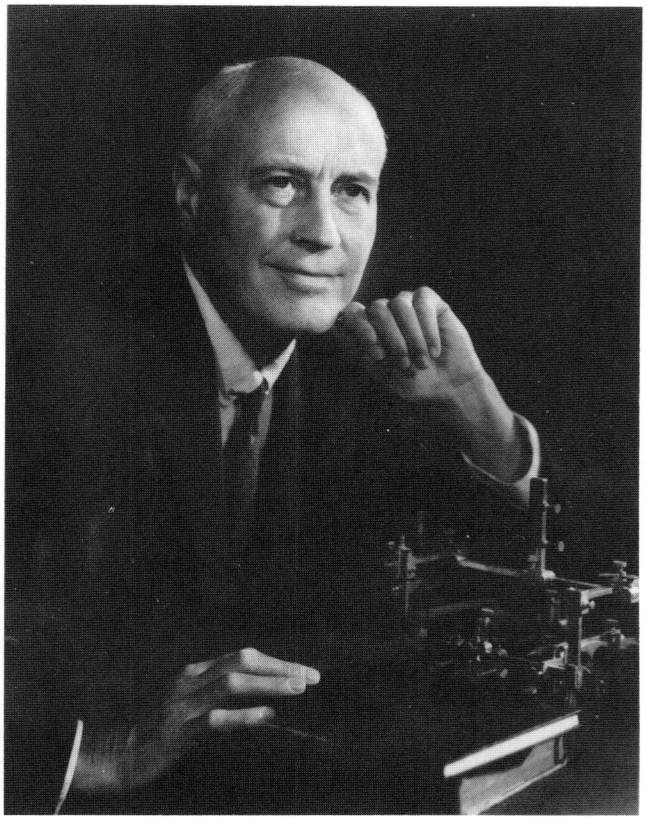

Magoun was personally involved in all of these studies, employing Ranson's newly commissioned reconstruction of a Horsley-Clarke stereotaxic instrument for making localized lesions and stimulating specific nuclei in the cat or monkey hypothalamus. He worked closely with Ingram and Fisher on cats in which supraoptic nucleus lesions led to diabetes insipidus presumably by denervating pituicytes, then considered the source of antidiuretic hormone. He also found that cutting the pituitary stalk at the median eminence level in monkeys induced polyuria and polydipsia while destroying the large nerve cells in the supraoptic nucleus by retrograde degeneration. He published these latter results in *Endocrinology* and *The Anatomical Record* in 1939.

In the cat studies there were observations that these same anterior hypothalamic lesions created problems in reproductive behavior, pregnancy, and parturition, the last probably attributable to the loss of neurohypophyseal oxytocin. These cats never came into heat and never bred in the laboratory. Magoun worked with Fisher, Dey and Brookhart in studying these problems in the guinea pig in which they induced persistent estrus and anestrus with differential lesions. He also collaborated with Philip Bard in a study in which electrolytic lesions in the female cat hypothalamus blocked estrous behavior in spite of estrogen injections, results which they reported in Bard's chapter in the 1940 volume 20 of Research Publications of the Association for Research in Nervous and Mental Disease entitled *The Hypothalamus*. In that memorable symposium, dedicated to Ranson, there were more references to Magoun than to any other person except Ranson himself. Interestingly, it should be pointed out that this same volume contained the classic proposal by neuroendocrine pioneers Ernst and Berta Scharrer, that posterior pituitary hormones might actually be produced by supraoptic neurons and delivered to the neurohypophysis by neurosecretion, a process now universally accepted as a basic concept in neuroendocrinology.

After Ranson's death in 1942 Magoun transferred to Northwestern's Department of Anatomy and performed the brilliant research for which he is now most famous:

FIG. 1. H. W. Magoun (1907-1991) From: Sawyer, C. H. "Anterior Pituitary Neural Control Concepts." In: Endocrinology: People and Ideas, edited by S. M. McCann. Bethesda, MD: American Physiological Society, 1988, chap 2, p 28 (The creditline was suggested by the American Physiological Society).

Received April 29, 1991.
"Remembrance" articles discuss people and events as remembered by the author. The opinion(s) expressed are solely those of the writer and do not reflect the view of the Journal or The Endocrine Society.

the elucidation of the role of the brainstem reticular formation in sleep wakefulness, awareness, and other aspects of higher nervous activity. This work won him many honors and awards including the Weinstein, Jacoby, Borden and Passano Awards as well as the Lashley and Gerard Prizes, the last as recently as 1989.

In 1950 Magoun accepted the chair of Anatomy in the new medical school at UCLA, and he soon started organizing an interdisciplinary institute patterned after Ranson's; it came to be known as the UCLA Brain Research Institute (BRI). Wanting neuroendocrinology to be strongly represented in his new institute, Magoun invited several young neuroendocrinologists to join him during the next few years. These included, chronologically, Charles Sawyer, Sidney Roberts, John Green, Robert Porter, Warner Florscheim, Karl Knigge, Charles Barraclough, John Pierce, Jessamine Hilliard, James Hayward, and Roger Gorski. During the last 35 years this neuroendocrine staff has been host to hundreds of visiting investigators from all over the world.

Magoun did not personally work on neuroendocrine projects at UCLA, but he inspired and promoted, by lectures, symposia, discussions, advice and encouragement, the search for involvement of the whole nervous system in controlling endocrine secretion and the feedback action of hormones on brain mechanisms and behavior. His broad comprehensive grasp of brain-endocrine interactions was captured in his 1963 monograph entitled, *The Waking Brain* (Charles C Thomas, Publisher). The BRI's Laboratory of Neuroendocrinology has continued to be active, and its current chief is Roger Gorski, who is also Chairman of the Department of Anatomy and Cell Biology. Magoun's sustained interest in and support of this laboratory will be sorely missed.

Charles Sawyer
Department of Anatomy
University of California-
 Los Angeles
School of Medicine

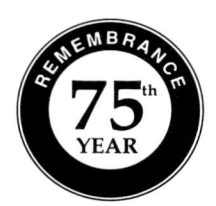

Remembrance Project: Origins of RIA

How did RIA begin? It was a serendipitous discovery in that it was a fallout from our investigations into what might be considered an unrelated study. Prompted by the suggestion of Dr. I. Arthur Mirsky that maturity-onset diabetes might not be due to an absolute deficiency of insulin secretion but rather to its abnormally rapid degradation by an enzyme which Mirsky called insulinase (1), Dr. Solomon A. Berson and I attempted to study the metabolism of ^{131}I-insulin after iv administration to diabetic and nondiabetic subjects (2). We observed a slower rate of disappearance of the ^{131}I-insulin from the plasma of subjects who had been treated with insulin whether or not they were diabetic. We postulated that the slower disappearance was a consequence of the binding of labeled insulin to antibodies that had developed in response to administration of foreign proteins-*i.e.* animal insulins. We used a variety of physicochemical systems, including, among others, paper electrophoresis, ultracentrifugal analysis, and salting out methods, to prove that the protein that bound insulin in the plasma of insulin-treated subjects had the characteristics of an antibody, an IgG immunoglobulin. This concept was not acceptable to immunologists of the mid-1950s. The original paper describing these findings was rejected by *Science* and initially rejected by the *Journal of Clinical Investigation* (JCI). The JCI letter of rejection was subsequently published in my Nobel Lecture (3). The paper was finally accepted after we omitted the words "insulin antibody" from the title (2) and documented our conclusion that the binding globulin was indeed an antibody by showing how it met the definition of antibody given in a standard textbook of bacteriology and immunity. To determine the concentration of antibody-binding sites in plasma we incubated labeled insulin and increasing concentrations of unlabeled insulin together with a fixed dilution of the antiserum. As the concentration of unlabeled insulin increased the amount of insulin bound to the antibody in the plasma increased although the fraction of labeled insulin bound to antibody decreased. While using this method to determine the maximum insulin-binding capacity of plasma antibody (2), we soon appreciated that the method could be used reciprocally to determine antigen (4, 5). Unfortunately with the human antisera then available to us, the sensitivity was not sufficient to determine circulating insulin in humans (5). However we did use this technique to follow the disappearance of beef-pork insulin administered iv to rabbits. Shortly thereafter we observed that antisera produced in guinea pigs immunized with animal insulins provided the requisite sensitivity and the assay of fasting and stimulated circulating insulin in man became possible (6, 7).

Our first discovery was that in newly discovered diabetic subjects there was a delay in insulin secretion in response to oral glucose administration. However in response to their sustained hyperglycemia during the test these patients became markedly hyperinsulinemic. Immediately after the publication of this paper (7) a large number of investigators requested the opportunity to visit our laboratory to learn immunoassay methodology. In response to these requests we organized a "Workshop on Insulin Immunoassay," held October 20-21, 1960, which had 43 attendees. Three additional immunoassay workshops attended by 85 participants were held in 1963, 1964, and 1965. Although only an occasional paper other than those from our laboratory appeared in prominent American journals of endocrinology and diabetes before 1965 (3), by the late 1960s RIA had become a major tool in endocrine laboratories around the world. A significant fraction of the flood of papers in the late 1960s was contributed by those who had attended our workshops.

RIA was first applied to the measurement of peptide hormones in plasma since it provided the specificity and sensitivity required to measure the minute concentrations of these substances (10^{-10}–10^{-12} M) in the presence of billion-fold higher concentrations of plasma proteins (8-12). Complications were introduced by an appreciation that several of the peptide hormones cross-reacting in an RIA system were present in the circulation in more than one form with different biological activities (13-15). The nonpeptidal hormones are present in plasma in considerably higher concentrations than the peptide hormones and RIA was soon applied to their measurement as well (16-18). RIA has since found application in the assay of a large variety of nonhormonal substances including viruses (19) and pharmacological agents (20). RIA and related immunoassays have since found application around the world in the measurement of hundreds of substances of biological interest.

Received May 31, 1991.

"Remembrance" articles discuss people and events as remembered by the author. The opinion(s) expressed are solely those of the writer and do not reflect the view of the Journal or The Endocrine Society.

Rosalyn S. Yalow
Solomon A. Berson Research Laboratory
Veterans Affairs Medical Center

References

1. Mirsky IA 1952 The etiology of diabetes mellitus in man. Recent Prog Horm Res 7:437–465
2. Berson SA, Yalow RS, Bauman A, Rothschild MA, Nuverly K 1956 Insulin-I^{131} metabolism in human subjects: demonstration of insulin binding globulin in the circulation of insulin treated subjects. J Clin Invest 35:170–190
3. Yalow RS 1978 Radioimmunoassay: a probe for the fine structure of biologic systems. Science 200:1236–1245
4. Berson SA, Yalow RS 1957 Kinetics of reaction between insulin and insulin-binding antibody. J Clin Invest 36:873
5. Berson SA 1957 In: Levine R, Anderson E (eds) Resume of Conference on Insulin Activity in Blood and Tissue Fluids. National Institute of Health, Bethesda, MD, May 9–10, p 7
6. Yalow RS, Berson SA 1959 Assay of plasma insulin in human subjects by immunological methods. Nature 184:1648–1649
7. Yallow RS, Berson SA 1960 Immunoassay of endogenous plasma insulin in man. J Clin Invest 38:1157–1175
8. Roth J, Glick SM, Yalow RS 1963 Hypoglycemia: a potent stimulus to secretion of growth hormone. Science 140:987–988
9. Utiger RD 1965 Radioimmunoassay of human plasma thyrotropin. J Clin Invest 44:1277–1286
10. Berson SA, Yalow RS 1968 Radioimmunoassay of ACTH in plasma. J Clin Invest 47:2725–2751
11. Saxena BB, Demura H, Gandy HM, Peterson RE 1968 Radioimmunoassay of human follicle stimulating and luteinizing hormones in plasma. J Clin Endocrinol Metab 28:519
12. Yalow RS, Berson SA 1970 Radioimmunoassay of gastrin. Gastroenterology 58:1–14
13. Berson SA, Yalow RS 1968 Immunochemical heterogeneity of parathyroid hormone in plasma. J Clin Endocrinol Metab 28:1037–1047
14. Roth J, Gorden P, Pastan I 1968 "Big insulin": a new component of plasma insulin detected by immunoassay. Proc Natl Acad Sci USA 61:138–145
15. Yalow RS, Berson SA 1970 Size and charge distinctions between endogenous human plasma gastrin in peripheral blood and heptadecapeptide gastrins. Gastroenterology 58:609–615
16. Chopra IJ 1972 A radioimmunoassay for measurement of thyroxine in unextracted serum. J Clin Endocrinol Metab 34:938–947
17. Chopra IJ, Solomon DH, Beall GN 1971 Radioimmunoassay for measurement of triiodothyronine in human serum. J Clin Invest 50:2033–2041
18. Abraham GE 1974 Radioimmunoassay of steroids in biological materials. In: Radioimmunoassay and Related Procedures in Medicine. II, International Atomic Energy Agency, Vienna, Austria, vol 2:3–28
19. Walsh JH, Yalow RS, Berson SA 1970 Detection of Australia antigen and antibody by means of radioimmunoassay techniques. J Infect Dis 121:550–554
20. Oliver Jr GC, Parker BM, Brasfield DL, Parker CW 1968 The measurment of digitoxin in human serum by radioimmunoassay. J Clin Invest 47:1035–1042

Henry Stanley Plummer

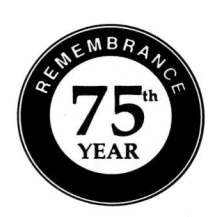

Henry Stanley Plummer, whose father was a country physician and whose mother was a schoolteacher, was born in 1874 in Hamilton, a small village twenty miles south of Rochester, Minnesota. While much interested in studying toward the engineering profession, he later decided on medicine. He graduated from Northwestern University Medical School in 1898, and returned to join his father's practice in Racine, Minnesota, a town near Rochester, where the family had moved in 1893.

At this time, Drs. William J. and Charles H. Mayo practiced medicine in Rochester in association with their father, Dr. William Worrall Mayo, and three other physicians. Henry Plummer's father, Dr. Albert Plummer, asked Dr. Will Mayo in 1900 to see a patient in consultation. When Dr. Mayo arrived with his horse and buggy at his destination, the elder Doctor Plummer was ill; so he asked his son to accompany Dr. Mayo to the patient's home. Henry carried his microscope, and on the way he conversed about the blood and its diseases. After he arrived, he made smears of the patient's blood, and showed that the patient had leukemia. He also made smears of the hired man's blood to demonstrate the marked differences between the normal blood and that of the patient. Dr. Mayo was greatly impressed by the young physician's brilliance and scientific approach to medical problems. When he returned home, he suggested to his brother that they invite Henry to join their association, which Dr. Plummer did, soon thereafter.

Since Rochester was located in the "center" of the goiter belt, Henry Plummer saw many patients with many types of goiter. Dr. Louis B. Wilson, a pathologist who joined the group, noted that for some patients who had thyroidectomy because of hyperthyroidism, the removed tissue was that of diffuse parenchymatous hypertrophy, while for others this was not so. By meticulous observation, Plummer determined that patients whose thyroids contained diffuse parenchymatous hypertrophy had Graves' disease (called exothalmic goiter), while those whose glands did not show parenchymatous hypertrophy had nodular goiters and no eye changes, characteristic nervous status, or tendency toward the development of crisis as seen in Graves' disease. He first reported

---

Received May 2, 1991.

"Remembrance," articles discuss people and events as remembered by the author. The opinion(s) expressed are solely those of the writer and do not reflect the view of the Journal or The Endocrine Society.

these observations in 1913 at a meeting of the American Medical Association; they were published in the same year in the *Journal of the American Medical Association*. At first, Plummer's views were not widely accepted by the medical community; but opinions soon recognized that "Plummer's disease" would become the eponym for hyperthyroidism with adenomatous (or nodular) goiter.

Mayo Clinic's Edward C. Kendall isolated thyroxine from the thyroid gland in 1914. Over the next few years, Plummer hypothesized that the disease of toxic, nodular goiter was simply caused by the overproduction of normal thyroxine by the nodule or nodules. In Grave's disease, by contrast, the cause was an excess production of an "abnormal" thyroxine, perhaps deficient in its iodine content. While iodine-containing substances had been used for centuries in treating goiters, thyroidologists in Plummer's time generally believed that iodine should not be given to patients with goiters. This opinion probably arose from reports of Kocher in Switzerland, and others, that euthyroid patients with endemic goiters who were treated with iodine would sometimes become hyperthyroid.

Graves' disease in Plummer's time was a very serious and sometimes fatal disorder. Plummer saw about 15 patients per year who arrived in thyroid crisis and died in spite of all treatment. Surgery on patients with Graves' disease sometimes involved risky procedures, usually resulting in a 3.5% mortality rate from postoperative thyroid crisis. Because of this, surgeons sometimes injected hot water into the thyroid or quickly ligated thyroid vessels with the hope of decreasing the toxic state before attempting thyroidectomy.

By 1922, Plummer had decided that the administration of iodine to patients who had hyperthyroidism due to Graves' disease might ameliorate the symptoms. Thus, in March 1922, he prescribed iodine in the form of Lugol's solution in 10 minim doses—once, twice, or three times per day—to patients with Graves' disease. He immediately noted a gratifyingly marked improvement in symptoms and a reduced level of the metabolic rate. Moreover, within 10 days of starting treatment with Lugol's solution, the patients safely underwent thyroid surgery. Plummer found that after the introduction of preoperative iodide treatment the surgical mortality dropped to under 1%. In addition, whereas between 1918 and 1922 there had been 75 nonoperative deaths due to

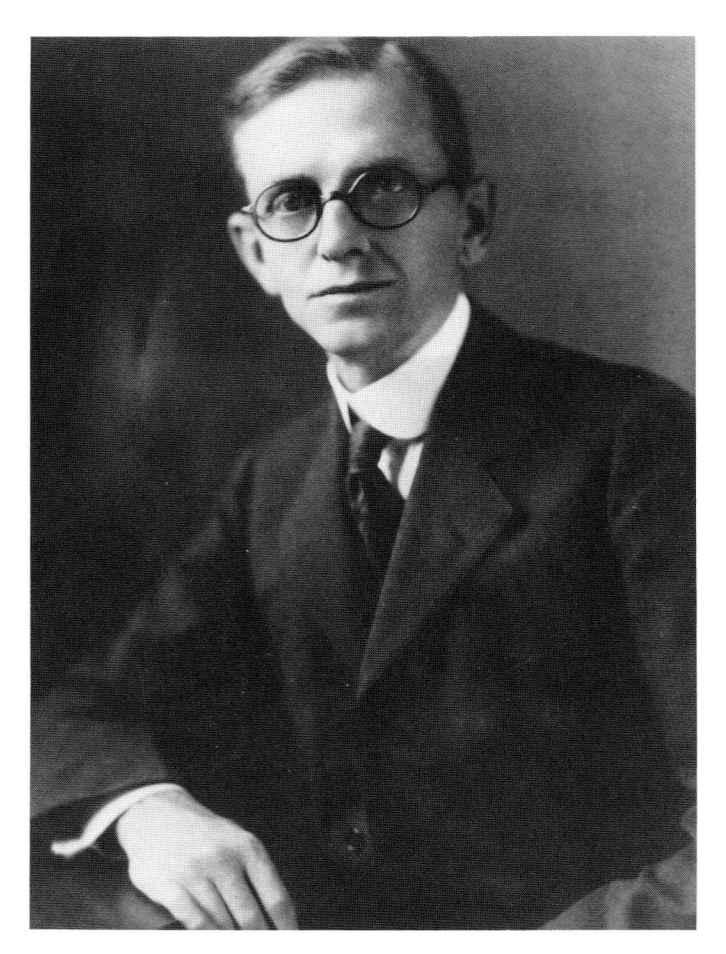

FIG. 1. Henry Stanley Plummer (1874–1936)

Graves' disease at the Mayo Clinic, in 1923 after the introduction of iodine use there was only one. Plummer reported these findings at meetings of both the Association of American Physicians and the Iowa State Medical Society, in 1923, and his announcement helped usher in the era of the great goiter surgeons.

Interest in the thyroid was not the only subject of interest which occupied Henry Plummer's time; he was a man of many talents. His first activity after joining the Mayo practice in 1901 was the development of a medical laboratory. Before this time, urinalysis and simple blood tests marked the main laboratory procedures. His next interest pursued the development of x-ray diagnosis and therapy, a completely new field, since roentgenography had only been discovered and described by Wilhelm Konrad Roentgen in 1895. Plummer pioneered in the use and modification of x-ray procedures, and developed, as did so many early workers with x-rays, radiation burns on his hands.

Dr. Plummer's practice drew him into the study of disease of the esophagus, including cardiospasm, diverticula, and stricture. Because lye solutions were often used for domestic needs, children and sometimes adults occasionally swallowed them. These accidents produced severe, acute inflammation of the esophagus, followed by ulceration and cicatricial obstruction. For the dilation of both cardiospasm and the constriction of lye burns, Plummer worked out a method of introducing the sound into the esophagus, guided by a previously swallowed, silk thread. Although he had not originated the concept of the hydrostatic dilator for such lesions, he pioneered its use in the midwest United States, and he made numerous modifications of the dilators in use. He also worked with the removal of foreign bodies from the bronchus and esophagus. Frequently, when he found he had no suitably designed instrument for removal of an object, he would make such an instrument in his well equipped workshop in his home. When he returned to the Clinic, he would amaze his surgical colleagues by the successful removal with his homemade instrument.

When Willem Einthoven (1860–1927) described electrocardiography and its usage between 1903 and 1906, Plummer realized its importance. He obtained one of the

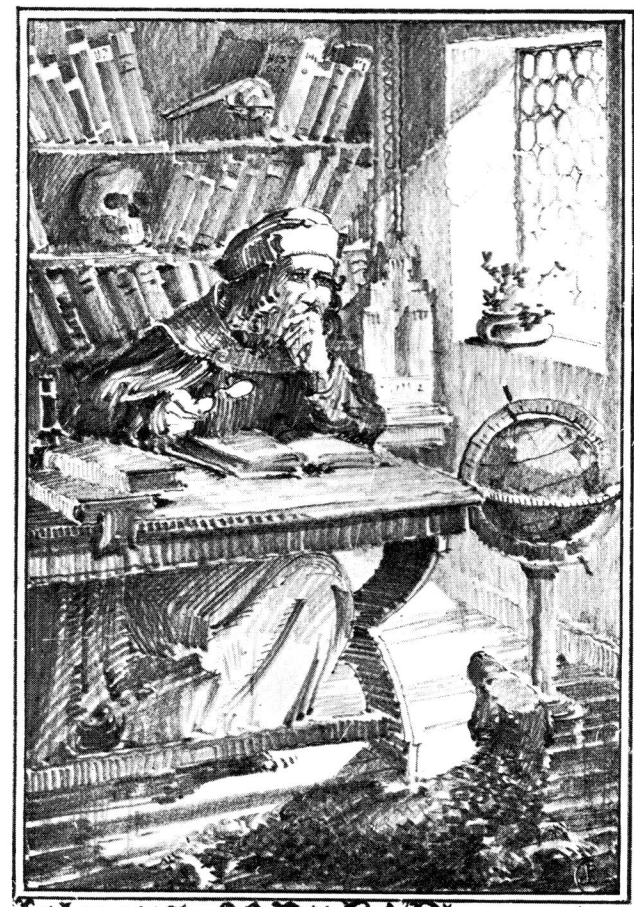

FIG. 2. Bookplate of Dr. Plummer's Rare Book Collection.

machines in 1914 and showed how to devise a string galvanometer to register electrical changes in the human heart, and to diagnose heart disorders. He greatly encouraged his associates to learn and use this innovative procedure.

Henry Plummer was solely responsible organizing and implementing the excellent filing system, record storage, and cross-indexing of patient records, which is still used today in the Mayo Clinic, with great success. This procedure was unique to the Rochester practice, because the patients' histories and findings were formerly recorded and stored in large ledgers, a most cumbersome method. But Plummer devised printed record sheets for individual patients so that the complete record for each could be stored in one packet.

Because of his special talents in engineering, mechanics, and architecture, he played a conspicuous, leading role in construction of new buildings on the Mayo campus. When it was decided in 1912 to construct a building for the use of the many members of the rapidly growing group, then called the Mayo Clinic, Plummer planned the room layout, the intra-Clinic communication system, special colored lights as signals above the doors of the examining rooms, and the central telephone office. He, again, was chiefly responsible for almost all of the design and planning of a 16-storied building, completed in 1929, to alleviate the pressing need for more adequate space. This building, named after him, is in full use today, and is an architectural and artistic gem. Plummer installed an intricate mechanical system for the transportation of patients' records and x-rays throughout the buildings. He also planned an extensive pedestrian-concourse subway system to interconnect the Mayo Clinic buildings and an adjacent hotel.

Late in the day on a December afternoon in 1936, Henry Plummer left the Clinic to be driven home. On the way he realized that he was having serious trouble, and he later told his wife at his bedside that he was having a cerebral thrombosis. Because he knew that he would soon become unconscious, he asked to see his family, once more. He saw them shortly before he lapsed into a coma, and died next day at the age of 62.

Dr. Plummer's collected works are located in the History of Medicine collection of the Mayo Medical Libraries and in the Archives of the Mayo Historical Unit. His letters and published papers and monographs reflect an unusual biobibliographical contribution to medical science. He was a brilliant man whom many described as a genius who lived far ahead of his time.

William M. McConahey
Professor Emeritus
Mayo Clinic
Donald S. Pady
History of Medicine Library
Mayo Foundation

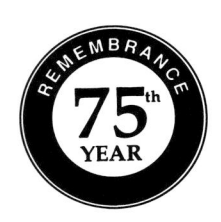

Remembrance of Dr. Alfred Jost

Dr. Alfred Jost died suddenly at his home, in the early morning of February 3, 1991, of a heart attack, at the age of 74. Just retired from the Collège de France, a prestigious school for higher education, he was still active in research, in spite of the demands made on his time by his duties as secretary of the French Academy of Science.

Dr. Jost is rightly regarded as the father of modern fetal endocrinology. Up to 1950, birds were the favorite embryological models, because of the technical accessibility of the avian egg. Jost was the first to apply surgical techniques to the intrauterine mammalian fetus. By castrating fetal rabbits at an early, ambivalent stage, he succeeded in preventing male differentiation: the genetic males were born with persistent Müllerian ducts and no Wolffian derivatives (1).

Were both effects due to the same cause? By comparing the effect on female fetal sex differentiation of an implanted testosterone crystal and a grafted testicular fragment, Alfred Jost proved the duality of fetal testicular secretin (Fig. 1) (2). In contrast to testicular tissue, testosterone was unable to induce the regression of the female sex primordia, and Jost logically concluded that another testicular hormone must be present to accomplish this task. He named this putative factor "l'hormone inhibitrice," in English the "Müllerian inhibitor." Paradoxically, this hypothesis was better received by physicians abroad than by his fellow scientists. Etienne Wolff and his school continued for many years to uphold the theory that testosterone alone was responsible for Müllerian regression (3)...

Through his brother, Dr. Marc Jost, who lived in Mexico City and was familiar with his experiments, Alfred Jost was invited to present his results at the First International Congress of Obstetrics and Gynecology, held in 1949 in Mexico City. On his return trip, he visited the Carnegie Institute in Washington, and one of the Embryology Associates, Dr. Robert K. Burns, suggested that he meet a clinician at Johns Hopkins, who was interested in human genital anomalies. One of Dr. Jost's favorite stories (4) was that of his first encounter with Dr. Lawson Wilkins. During a whole afternoon, the founder of pediatric endocrinology confronted the young Frenchman with cases of abnormal sex differentiation, Turner's syndrome, congenital adrenal hyperplasia, testicular feminization, and asked how the theory of the duality of fetal testicular secretion could explain the clinical picture. At the end of the day, Wilkins said: "I'm convinced!" He then undertook to "market" the Jost theory among American endocrinologists. The Nobel prize winners Gregory Pincus and Bernardo Houssay, followed by Howard W. Jones Jr., Melvin Grumbach, Maria New, Claude Migeon, to name only a few, became his fervent admirers and warm personal friends.

An intellectual giant, Dr. Jost did not neglect the technical aspect of laboratory investigation. "Everyone can have ideas," he liked to say, "not everyone can carry them out." It took him a year and a half of hard work to successfully carry out the castration of fetal rabbits, (Fig. 2) and his technical difficulties were not alleviated by the fact that in hungry postwar Paris, rabbits were easier to obtain for the kitchen than for the laboratory. Having demonstrated the role of the fetal testis in sex differentiation, Jost developed another original technique to study its pituitary regulation. Knowing that some acephalic human fetuses had been described, he decided to try decapitating rabbit fetuses. The first three died, but the fourth survived several days, judging from its size. Later, encephalectomy was devised to remove the hypothalamus, while leaving the pituitary *in situ*. Fetal decapitation and encephalectomy became routine techniques in Jost's laboratory and were applied to the study of pituitary regulation of various organs: the testis (5), the thyroid (6), the adrenals (7), and the liver (8).

However, sex differentiation always remained Jost's favorite subject. He devoted significant efforts to the study of freemartininism, and was the first to suggest that the ovarian aplasia and masculinization observed in female fetuses joined to male twins by placental anastomoses could be due to the factor responsible for Müllerian regression (9). Efforts to isolate the Müllerian inhibitor were initiated in his laboratory by Régine Picon: she showed that the fetal rat Müllerian duct, explanted in the absence of gonads at day-14 postcoitum, was a reliable and convenient target organ for testing anti-Müllerian activity (10). The Müllerian inhibitor, now called anti-Müllerian hormone, Müllerian-inhibiting substance or factor, was characterized as a glycoprotein dimer (11), purified from calf fetal testes (12) and culture medium

---

Received May 29, 1991.

"Remembrance," articles discuss people and events as remembered by the author. The opinion(s) expressed are solely those of the writer and do not reflect the view of the Journal or The Endocrine Society.

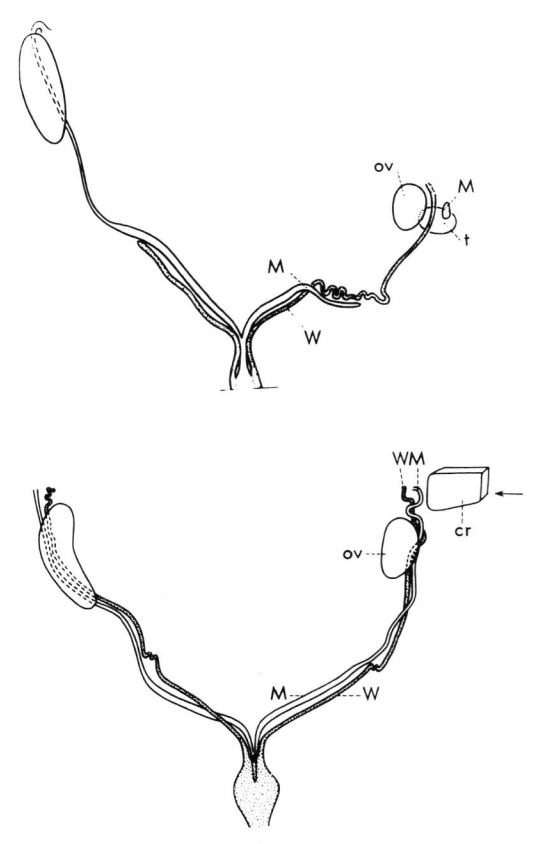

FIG. 1. Graphic reconstruction (slightly schematized) of genital tract of two female rabbit fetuses 28 days old. *Top*, Fetal testis (t) was grafted near ovary (ov) on day 20. Partial inhibition of Müllerian duct (M) and partial maintenance of Wolffian duct (W, stippled) resulted. *Bottom*, Crystal of testosterone propionate (cr) was implanted near ovary on day 20. There was maintenance of Wolffian ducts and no inhibition of the Müllerian ducts (from 20, with permission).

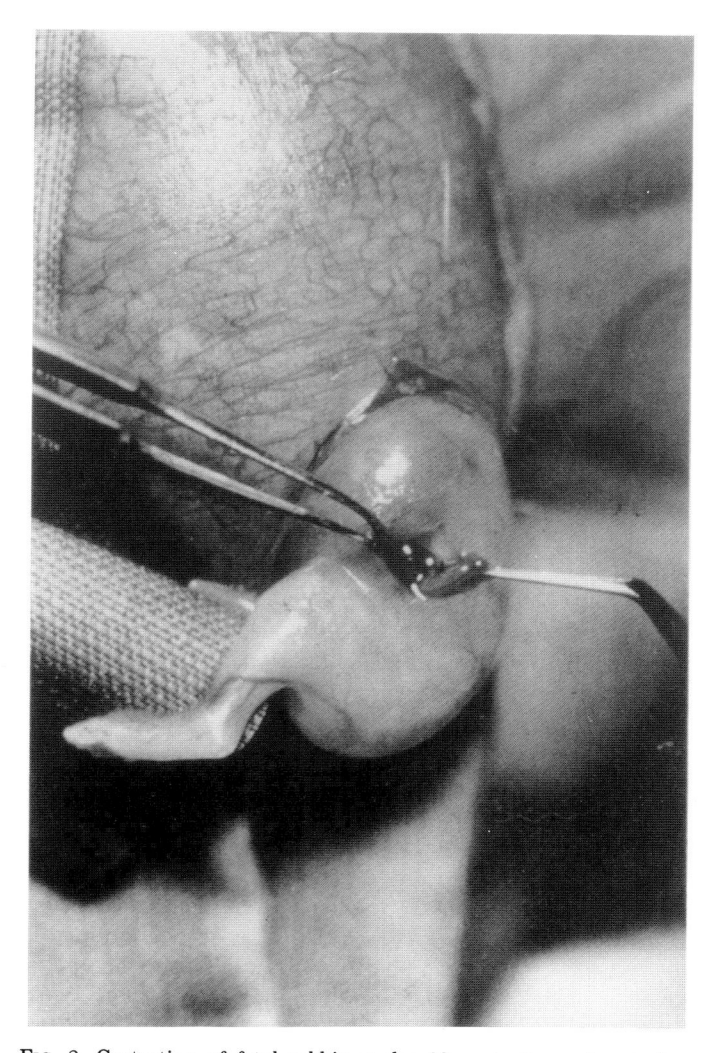

FIG. 2. Castration of fetal rabbit at day-23 postcoïtum. An uterine chamber has been opened, the posterior end of the fetus is exteriorized, its flank incised and the testis and mesonephros are exposed. After testicular resection, the fetus is replaced into the uterus. For practical reasons, the operation has been photographed using a fetus past the ambisexual stage, castration at that age would not be expected to result in female sex differentiation. From Ref. 19, with permission.

of transfected cells in culture (13), cloned (14), and localized on the human genome (15). A member of the TGF-β family (14, 16), the hormone is now detectable by enzyme-linked immunosorbent assay in human serum (17) and a transgenic mouse line expressing human Müllerian inhibitor under the control of a heterologous promoter has been constructed (18). Jost's interest in his "baby's" progress never wavered, and is reflected in his last manuscript, published after his death (19).

Dr. Jost's many admirers will be stunned to learn that this great scientist was initially destined to become a grocer's assistant. Young Alfred's father died when he was 13, and a year later, his mother became unable to care for her four sons. The two older boys were supporting themselves, the youngest was farmed out to his grandmother and Madame Jost was making arrangements with a grocer to employ Alfred, when Madame Oguse, a neighbor in the same building, touched by the boy's predicament, offered to raise him with her own children. André Oguse, a professor of ancient Greek at the University of Strasbourg, struck with the child's keen intelligence, tutored him so that the same year he rose from the bottom to the top of his class and, in 1936, was admitted to the prestigious Ecole Normale Supérieure. Alfred's intellectual preoccupations did not however blind him to his surroundings: he fell head over heels in love with the young daughter of the house. When they were married in 1940, Christiane was 16. Their union lasted more than 50 years.

Dr. Jost's pioneering contribution to developmental endocrinology ensures him an everlasting place in the scientific Pantheon. He will remain alive in the heart of those who had the privilege of knowing this great man. It is difficult, particularly for someone for whom English

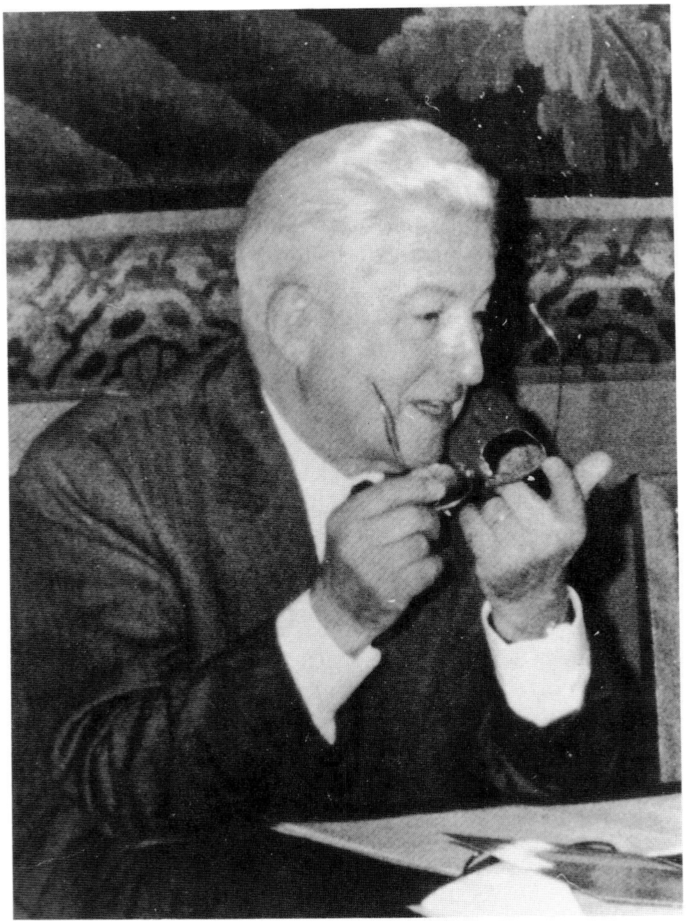

FIG. 3. Professor Alfred Jost

is not a native language, to find the words to describe his simplicity, his genuine interest in young people, his intellectual honesty, and the charm and authority which radiated from his person. In this picture taken at a meeting (Fig. 3), he seems about to speak. How hard it is for those who loved him to believe they will never hear his voice again...

Nathalie Josso
Unité de Recherches sur l'Endocrinologie
  du Développement INSERM
Ecole Normale Supérieure
Montrouge, France

References

1. Jost A 1947 Recherches sur la différenciation sexuelle de l'embryon de lapin. III. Rôle des gonades foetales dans la différenciation sexuelle somatique. Arch Anat Microsc Morphol Exp 36:271–315
2. Jost A 1953 Problems of fetal endocrinology: the gonadal and hypophyseal hormones. Rec Progr Horm Res 8:379–418
3. Lutz-Ostertag Y 1976 Nouvelles preuves de l'action de la testostérone sur le développement des canaux de Müller de l'embryon d'Oiseau en culture in vitro. CR Acad Sci Série D Paris 278:2351–2353
4. Jost A 1972 A new look at the mechanisms controlling sex differentiation in mammals. Johns Hopkins Med J 130:38–53
5. Jost A 1951 Recherches sur la différenciation sexuelle de l'embryon de Lapin IV. Organogenèse sexuelle masculine après décapitation du foetus. Arch Anat Microsc Morphol Exp 40:247–281
6. Jost A 1953 Sur le développement de la thyroïde chez le foetus de Lapin décapité. Arch Anat Microsc Morphol Exp 42:168–183
7. Jost A, Cohen A 1966 Signification de l'"atrophie" des surrénales foetales du Rat provoquée par l'hypophysectomie (décapitation). Dev Biol 14:154–168
8. Jost A, Jacquot R 1954 Recherches sur le contrôle hormonal de la charge en glycogène du foie foetal du Lapin et du Rat. CR Acad Sci série D Paris 239:98–100
9. Jost A, Vigier B, Prépin J 1972 Freemartins in cattle: the first steps of sexual organogenesis. J Reprod Fertil 29:349–379
10. Picon R 1969 Action du testicule foetal sur le développement in vitro des canaux de Müller chez le rat. Arch Anat Microsc Morphol Exp 58:1–19
11. Picard JY, Tran D, Josso N 1978 Biosynthesis of labeled anti-Müllerian hormone by fetal testes: evidence for the glycoprotein nature of the hormone and for its disulfide-bonded structure. Mol Cell Endocrinol 12:17–30
12. Picard JY, Josso N 1984 Purification of testicular anti-Müllerian hormone allowing direct visualization of the pure glycoprotein and determination of yield and purification factor. Mol Cell Endocrinol 34:23–29
13. Wallen J, Cate RL, Kiefer DM, Riemen MW, Martinez D, Hoffman RM, Donahoe PK, Von Hoff DD, Pepinsky B, Oliff A 1989 Minimal anti-proliferative effect of recombinant Müllerian inhibiting substance on gynecological tumor cell lines and tumor explants. Cancer Res 49:2005–2011
14. Cate RL, Mattaliano RJ, Hession C, Tizard R, Farber NM, Cheung A, Ninfa EG, Frey AZ, Gash DJ, Chow EP, Fisher RA, Bertonis JM, Torres G, Wallner BP, Ramachandran KL, Ragin RC, Manganaro TF, MacLaughlin DT, Donahoe PK 1986 Isolation of the bovine and human genes for müllerian inhibiting substance and expression of the human gene in animal cells. Cell 45:685–698
15. Cohen-Haguenauer O, Picard JY, Mattei MG, Serero S, Nguyen VC, de Tand MF, Guerrier D, Hors-Cayla MC, Josso N, Frézal J 1987 Mapping of the gene for anti-Müllerian hormone to the short arm of human chromosome 19. Cytogenet Cell Genet 44:2–6
16. Pepinsky RB, Sinclair LK, Chow EP, Mattaliano RJ, Manganaro TF, Donahoe PK, Cate RL 1988 Proteolytic processing of Müllerian inhibiting substance produces a transforming growth factor-β-like fragment. J Biol Chem 263:18961–18965
17. Miller WL 1990 Immunoassays for human mullerian inhibitory factor (MIF)—new insights into the physiology of MIF. J Clin Endocrinol Metab 70:8–10
18. Behringer RR, Cate RL, Froelick GJ, Palmiter RD, Brinster RL 1990 Abnormal sexual development in transgenic mice chronically expressing Müllerian inhibiting substance. Nature 345:167–170
19. Jost A 1991 Les péripéties d'une recherche: l'étude de la différenciation sexuelle. Med Sci 7:264–275
20. Jost A 1955 La biologie des androgènes chez l'embryon. In: IIIe Réunion des Endocrinologistes de Langue Française. Paris: Masson, pp 160–180

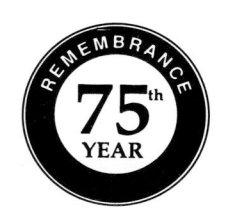

The Early Days of Steroid Radioimmunoassays at the Worcester Foundation

In the late 1960s, the Worcester Foundation for Experimental Biology in Shrewsbury, Massachusetts continued to maintain its position as a veritable "Mecca" of steroid research. The faculty included Drs. A. and H. Brodie, Burstein, Caspi, Chang, Lloyd, McCracken, Peron, Romanoff, S. and J. Tait, Townsley, Williams, and others. Postdoctoral training programs in Steroid Biochemistry and in Reproductive Biology were thriving, a distillation plant was producing "in house" organic solvents of chromatographic grade, and TLC, Bush I, and Bush II were parts of the vocabulary. The "double isotope" and "protein binding" assays were in routine use for quantitation of steroid hormones in biological fluids. At the same time, Dr. Guy Abraham was laboring in a one-person laboratory on an idea of devising a radioimmunoassay for estradiol. Unless I am mistaken, most of the biochemists and "mainstream" steroid workers were giving this project a probability of success which was not significantly different from zero. However, Guy was about to prove everyone wrong with his success in developing a solid-phase radioimmunoassay system for estradiol-17β (1).

At about the same time, a group of young scientists associated with the training programs was busy immunizing animals with various steroid conjugates in an attempt to interfere with hormone action by active and passive immunization and to develop radioimmunoassays. This group consisted of Drs. Burton Caldwell, Rex Scaramuzzi, Steven Tillson, and Ian Thorneycroft. Their efforts were singularly successful with a string of exciting papers appearing in various journals, and radioimmunoassays for progesterone, testosterone, and androstenedione becoming a reality in rapid succession. This was soon followed by a report at an opening session of The 1971 Endocrine Society Meeting of successful development of RIA for prostaglandin F_{2a} (2). The pace of progress in this group was rapid and publication of the various methods often lagged behind. Also, there seemed to be little concern for establishing a written record of who should receive credit for development of these procedures, and exactly when the various assays were first developed. In the meantime, Burt Caldwell, who headed this group, and his colleagues were wonderfully open about their work and not only willingly shared the antisera and assay protocols with whoever was interested, but publicized availability of the new assays and offered assistance in establishing them in other laboratories. As a result, some of these procedures were first described in publications from laboratories that did not participate in their development [e.g. testosterone RIA (3)]. Similarly, the critical role of Dr. Sumner Burstein who synthesized steroid conjugates (I believe mostly BSA-oximes and hemi-succinates) for these studies, or help provided by Drs. Tom Wittstruck and Ken Williams with magnetic resonance analysis and organic chemistry, would probably not be obvious from reading the literature.

Performance of the newly developed radioimmunoassays elicited a mixture of awe and incredulity. Not only were these procedures more sensitive than the previously available methods, but they were much less labor intensive and easier to learn. However, occasional difficulties with blank values or column chromatography tended to reinforce the suspicion that this new "magic" may be too good to be true. Hence, both the developers and the early users of these assays spent much time and energy on testing, validating, and comparing the results to those obtained by established methods. It was felt that chromatographic preparation of the sample was a must and the possibility of doing assays on unextracted serum or plasma was not even considered. Now, nearly 20 years later, this period seems very remote indeed. Radioimmunoassays for steroids are "routine" to the point that many manuscripts limit description of these procedures to quoting a single reference from another laboratory!

Obviously the Worcester Foundation was not the only place where steroid radioimmunoassays were being successfully developed. However, I believe that the impact of the procedures developed at this institution on the progress of endocrinology was remarkable. For many years, acknowledgments of Drs. Caldwell, Thorneycroft, and Abraham as providers of antisera appeared in what must have been hundreds of papers and there is little

---

Received July 10, 1991.

"Remembrance," articles discuss people and events as remembered by the author. The opinion(s) expressed are solely those of the writer and do not reflect the view of the Journal or The Endocrine Society.

NOTE: This brief assay is a personal view from an observer of a particular stage of steroid research at one institution. No attempt was made to provide a comprehensive review or to give credit to all those who provided help, financial support, and facilities for these studies.

doubt that a significant proportion of the world's literature dealing with reproductive endocrinology in the 1970s reported results of studies performed with the use of these reagents. I had a supply of Burt Caldwell's antiserum to testosterone until 1985!

In the present era of commercial RIA labs, easy-to-use kits, and sophisticated mathematical analysis of hormone levels measured in hundreds of serially collected samples, it is interesting to realize that as recently as 20 years ago measurements of steroid hormones were far from routine and it was exciting to be able to measure steroids in the amount of blood that could be collected from a mouse or a juvenile rat.

Andrzej Bartke
Professor and Chairman
Department of Physiology
Southern Illinois University School of Medicine

References

1. Abraham GA 1969 Solid-phase radioimmunoassay of estradiol-17$_\beta$. J Clin Endocrinol Metab 29:866–870
2. Caldwell BV, Brock WA, Burstein S, Speroff L, Radioimmunoassay of prostaglandin F$_{2\alpha}$. Program of the 53rd Annual Meeting of The Endocrine Society, San Francisco, CA, A-46, 1971 (Abstract 8)
3. Bartke A, Steele RE, Musto N, Caldwell BW 1973 Fluctuations in plasma testosterone levels in adult male rats and mice. Endocrinology 91:1223–1228

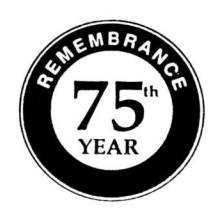

The Beginnings of an Endocrinologist

During my graduate studies I never had courses in endocrinology and pharmacology. Expressions such as "dose-response," "desensitization," "agonist/antagonist," in fact, all expressions relating to physiology were alien to my ears. I was a biochemist bred to believe in the reductionist philosophy of science, still much in vogue today. Grind, extract, purify, and reconstruct were the keys words in my lexicon. Nature, in all its mystery, was at my feet waiting to be dismembered into its constitutive parts and, as with any organic chemistry problem, reassembled as proof of one's unerring biochemical skills. That philosophy for me was dramatically altered several years later when I attempted to investigate whether fat cells were the source of lipoprotein lipase present in adipose tissue. I discovered that fat cells, which float because of their fat content, could be isolated from other cells by treatment with commercial preparations of collagenase (1). The fat cells contained lipoprotein lipase. My good fortune was that Bernardo Houssay, the great Argentine physiologist and Nobel Laureate was visiting my lab the day of the first successful experiment. "How do you know these are viable cells?", he queried. "Of course they are, just look under the microscope," I replied. "No," he said, "I will not be satisfied unless you can demonstrate that they are subject to the actions of hormones, such as insulin, that are known to act on adipose tissue." Down the hall I went to ask Sid Chernick and Bob Scow how to determine the actions of insulin. Two days later I had devised a means of collecting radioactive CO_2 released by the metabolism of glucose-1-^{14}C and demonstrated that insulin strikingly increased the amount released. I was nonplussed. Dr. Houssay was ecstatic. Apparently, this was the first demonstration that insulin acts on individual cells. Practically overnight I had become an endocrinologist; of sorts, that is. It was the guidance and inspiration of Robert Williams, the head of the Department of Endocrinology at the University of Washington, who inspired me to rethink my strategies in exploring the living process. No more grinding, extraction, and purification. Treatment of cells with phospholipases and other enzymes, preparation of fat cell "ghosts," and purification of cell membranes were the cautious, step-by-step means of exploring at what level of cell dismemberment insulin's actions remained. By 1967 I knew that the plasma membrane had to be the initiating site of action, but there my investigative prowess ended. The next momentous change for me came when Sutherland lectured at NIH about the enzyme adenyl cyclase (now adenylate or adenylyl cyclase). Aided by an assay of the enzyme's activity developed by Gopal Krishna, Lutz Birnbaumer, my first post-doc, and I discovered that the adenyl cyclase system in rat adipocytes was activated by several different hormones, acting through distinctive receptors, on what appeared to be a common enzyme (2). Moreover, the hormones increased the affinity of the system for Mg ions (3). Intrigued by these findings, we considered it likely that there is some common, Mg-dependent element that intervened between the receptors and enzyme and which could accommodate a system having so many "angels on a pinhead." At this point, Oscar Hechter entered into my life with long, wonderful discussions about cybernetics. Out of this came the transduction model of hormone action (4). Experimental evidence for the model came when Michiel Krans, while studying the binding of ^{125}I-glucagon to purified rat liver plasma membranes found that glucagon binding was a slow process that was essentially irreversible, in contrast to the rapid and reversible effects of the hormone on adenyl cyclase activity found by Lutz Birnbaumer and Steve Pohl. But the medium used for the hormone-binding studies was devoid of most of the ingredients employed for the adenyl cyclase studies. By the standard biochemical technique of adding and deleting each of the ingredients, we found that ATP was the culprit. However, I knew from experience in my graduate studies that one cannot rely on the purity of commercial ATP. We tested every known purine and pyrimidine nucleotide and subsequently discovered that GTP affected the binding of glucagon to its receptors and, as importantly, was necessary for glucagon to activate adenyl cyclase (5, 6). Since those discoveries more than 20 yr ago, transduction has become a key concept for explaining the actions of hormones and drugs on membrane processes. But, as I have learned over these many years, nature cannot simply be fathomed by knowing its chemical and physical composition. The living process has evolved far beyond our knowledge of physics and chemistry. Understanding the organization and integration of

---

Received May 22, 1991.

"Remembrance" articles discuss people and events as remembered by the author. The opinion(s) expressed are solely those of the writer and do not reflect the view of the Journal or The Endocrine Society.

all cellular information processing systems presents challenges that certainly will not be met in my lifetime, and perhaps never. But, at the very least, I have become, if not officially, at least in practise a full-fledged endocrinologist.

Martin Rodbell
Chief, Section on Signal Transduction
NIEHS-NIH

References

1. Rodbell M 1964 The metabolism of isolated fat cells. I. Effects of hormones on glucose metabolism and lipolysis. J Biol Chem 239:375–380
2. Birnbaumer L, Pohl SL, Rodbell M 1969 Adenyl cyclase in fat cells. I. Properties and the effects of adrenocorticotropin and fluoride. J Biol Chem 244:3468–3476
3. Birnbaumer L, Rodbell M 1969 Adenyl cyclase in fat cells. II. Hormone receptors. J Biol Chem 244:3477–3482
4. Rodbell M, Birnbaumer L, Pohl SL, Krans HMJ, Hormones, Receptors, and the Adenyl Cyclase System. Fogarty International Center Proceedings, Bethesda, MD, 1969:59–76
5. Rodbell M, Krans HMJ, Pohl SL, Birnbaumer L 1971 The glucagon-sensitive adenyl cyclase system in plasma membranes of rat liver. IV. Effects of guanyl nucleotides on binding of 125I-glucagon. J Biol Chem 246:1872–1876
6. Rodbell M, Birnbaumer L, Pohl SL, Krans HMJ 1971 The glucagon-sensitive system in plasma membranes of rat liver. V. An obligatory role of guanyl nucleotides in glucagon action. J Biol Chem 246:1877–1882

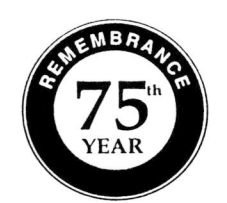

Peptide and Protein Hormones—from Biological Definitions to Chemical Compounds

Endocrinology to remember—how the application of new means for the purification and analysis of proteins led in the late 1940s and 1950s to the final establishment that the biological activity of some hormones (as well as enzymes) resides in simple peptides or proteins of defined amino acid sequence. Thus, though both insulin and urease had been crystallized in 1926, lingering doubts by some persisted well into the 1930s as to the true chemical nature of various biologically active principles. The picture changed dramatically in the next two decades and I was privileged to participate, with many others, in one major effort. The research concerned the active principles responsible for the uterine contracting, milk ejecting pressor, and antidiuretic activities of extracts of the posterior pituitary gland. Two hormones, oxytocin and vasopressin, were isolated; their covalent structure determined, and their chemical synthesis achieved.

The laboratory was that of Professor Vincent du Vigneaud and colleagues at Cornell University Medical College, New York. Dr. du Vigneaud was a superb bioorganic chemist whose interest in oxytocin and vasopressin (ADH) stemmed from his earlier work on the chemistry of insulin, which had been found, after its purification and crystallization, to be a sulfur-containing substance. It is difficult now to realize that for some years after the clinical usefulness of insulin was well established uncertainty remained as to whether the hormonal activity of even crystalline preparations was due to the absorption on the protein of an unknown hormonally active substance or an intrinsic property of a simple protein. Many amorphous insulin preparations contained significant amounts of a hyperglycemic activity later to be isolated and named glucagon. However, crystalline insulin was sufficiently homogeneous to permit Sanger's brilliant determination of the amino acid sequences of the insulin A and B chains. In Sanger's work ingenious use of partial hydrolysis and paper chromatography to prepare and analyze peptide fragments from each chain resulted in a unique solution for the sequences. Sanger's contribution to protein chemistry cannot be overestimated; it was the first to show that a protein was a definite compound with a precise covalent structure. An interesting aspect of the insulin work was that the methods of peptide separation and analysis were not quantitative, though the amino acid composition had been laboriously determined *inter alia* by Chibnall and associates with considerable precision. Insulin's molecular weight, however, was uncertain.

With the posterior pituitary hormones both purification and analysis were needed and, by pleasant coincidence, new techniques ideal for the problem were being developed at the Rockefeller Institute immediately adjacent to Cornell Medical College. One was the development by Lyman Craig of a method of purification involving a discontinuous extraction process which he called countercurrent distribution. In theory the process is the same as fractional distillation or many types of column chromatography. Craig's method proved ideal both for the separation and analysis of the extent of separation for small peptides and small proteins. It was used by him with particular success in showing that some peptide antibiotics, previously purified by fractional crystallization, were mixtures of closely related molecules. One important advantage of the technique was that recoveries are complete and analysis of the distribution patterns allows estimation of purity. Just a few laboratories away, Stanford Moore and William Stein were developing their chromatographic methods (first with starch, then with ion-exchange columns) for rapid and quantitative amino acid analysis of proteins. Because of the cordial scientific interchange between du Vigneaud and the Rockefeller scientists, I was able to apply quickly Moore and Stein's starch column methods for amino acid analysis of an unknown protein or peptide, namely the oxytocin of high biological activity purified by Livermore and du Vigneaud by means of countercurrent distribution. The first experiments clearly demonstrated the oxytocin preparation to contain only eight amino acids in equimolar amounts with only traces of other amino acids present. Total confirmation of composition and structure came with the chemical synthesis by du Vigneaud and others

---

Received July 27, 1991.

"Remembrance" articles discuss people and events as remembered by the author. The opinion(s) expressed are solely those of the writer and do not reflect the view of the Journal or The Endocrine Society.

Many scientists and laboratories contributed to the events summarized herein. For more detail see Sanger F 1988 Sequences, sequences, sequences. Annu Rev Biochem 57:1 and du Vigneau V 1960 Experiences in the polypeptide field: insulin to oxytocin. Ann N Y Acad Sci 88:537. Selected original papers can be found in Pierce JG (ed) 1982 Peptide and Protein Hormones. Hutchinson Ross, Stroudsburg, PA.

in 1953. Similar results with vasopressin followed in due course. One of my most pleasant recollections is of an early amino acid analysis of what was the best vasopressin (ADH) preparation then available in which a number of amino acids were found to predominate but with appreciable amounts of others present. Somewhat facetiously I placed a prediction of an octapeptide composition for vasopressin in my desk; a year later after the purification of highly active vasopressin by countercurrent distribution had been accomplished, the prediction was found to be correct. Such was the power of rapid quantitative amino acid analysis of a small peptide when combined with good luck. Pure vasopressin was obtained in 1951 and chemical synthesis of both hormones was achieved in 1952 and 1953. I was spending a year in F. G. Young's laboratory in Cambridge, England, investigating by countercurrent distribution whether GH activity was a property of a small peptide or of a larger protein then thought to have a mol wt of 44,000. It was not a small peptide. Interestingly enough, another hormone ACTH whose peptide nature was then not clear was being successfully separated from protein in Cambridge by use of the ion-exchange chromatographic methods of Stein and Moore by Dixon, Moore, Stack-Dunne, and Young. Back in New York the use of countercurrent distribution by Harfenist and Craig conclusively yielded the final bit of information necessary to determine the amino acid sequence of insulin, namely that the monomer mol wt was approximately 6,000 rather than 12,000.

Thus, in the 10 yr after World War II a number of excellent techniques were developed and used in the study of proteins not by physical means but by the approach of organic chemists. Good fortune also was present. Oxytocin and vasopressin turned out to be small peptides and the A and B chains of insulin contained only 21 and 30 amino acids, respectively. Application of the techniques to proteins at the other end of the molecular weight range such as thyroglobulin would not have been so successful. The purification of many hormonally active proteins and peptides then proceeded with such increasing rapidity that it is difficult to recall that in the mid-1940s only three naturally occurring peptides had been well characterized and their structures determined; how many are there now?

John G. Pierce
Professor Emeritus, Department of Biological Chemistry
UCLA School of Medicine—Los Angeles

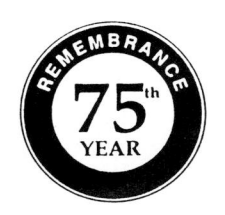

A Footnote to Pituitary Transplantation Research

It was by good fortune that Jack DeGroot visited my laboratory one Saturday morning during the mid-1950s. The visit could not have come at a more appropriate time, for he was skilled in the transtemporal surgical approach to the basal hypothalamus of the rat brain. Jack had formerly trained with Geoffrey Harris in the Department of Physiology, University of Cambridge, during the period when Harris perfected transtemporal surgery for his famous work on the pituitary stalk and the pituitary portal vessels.

In 1954 and 1956 I demonstrated that transplantation of the anterior pituitary gland away from its connection to the brain to a site in the renal capsule favored chronic secretion of PRL ("luteotrophin") whereas other trophic secretions were essentially lost. It was already known through the study by Harris and Jacobsohn that if anterior pituitaries were grafted near the pituitary stalk soon after hypophysectomy, normal ovarian functions resumed because of prompt regeneration of the portal vessels. In light of that information it seemed reasonable to propose that gonadotropic secretion from a pituitary graft, deficient after the gland had been on the kidney for several weeks, might be revived by retransplantation of the graft near the original site.

In 1955, Miroslava Nikitovitch-Winer chose to work in my laboratory on research for her Ph.D. dissertation. Among several projects involving pituitary transplantation and corpus luteum function she undertook the retransplantation experiment. The transtemporal route to the median eminence appeared to be the choice. As I recall, she made a considerable number of trials according to Harris' published description of the delicate surgery, but with elusive success in spite of increasing familiarity with the region. It was at that time that Jack DeGroot paid us his visit.

The two of them sat across the table from each other, while Jack with only words and his hands conjured up a much enlarged abstraction of the operative scene, detailing step by step the entire procedure of the transtemporal surgery. There was much discussion, of course. The upshot of the interchange was impressive: further attempts at the experiment were almost uniformly successful. The role that chance encounters can play in the progress of science can hardly be better illustrated.

The successful experiments demonstrated not only that the twice-damaged pituitary graft rapidly recovered its cyclic gonadotropic secretions upon return to hypothalamic control, but that thyrotropic and adrenocorticotropic secretions returned as well. Equally significant was the finding that the steady secretion of PRL, uninhibited while the graft was on the kidney, was diminished to levels compatible with the estrous cycles.

Jack DeGroot is now Professor Emeritus of Anatomy at the University of California School of Medicine, San Francisco. Miroslava B. Nikitovitch-Winer is Professor and Chairperson of the Department of Anatomy and Neurobiology, University of Kentucky Medical Center, Lexington.

John W. Everett
Professor Emeritus, Department of Neurobiology
Duke University Medical Center

Received June 20, 1991.

"Remembrance" articles discuss people and events as remembered by the author. The opinion(s) expressed are solely those of the writer and do not reflect the view of the Journal or The Endocrine Society.

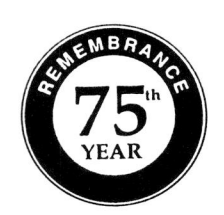

The Long and Evans Monograph on the Estrous Cycle in the Rat

This 1922 monograph (1) described for the first time with precision, accuracy, and detail the estrous cycle of this hardy, rapidly reproducing laboratory animal. It thus laid the foundation for its subsequent use in the isolation and characterization not only of ovarian hormones but also of hypophyseal gonadotropic hormones. Both authors were members of the University of California faculty in Berkeley, Long since 1908 and Evans since 1915. Long was a Ph.D. (1908) from Harvard where his doctoral dissertation under Prof. E. L. Mark had been on the maturation of the egg of the mouse, clearly the beginning of his work on reproductive physiology. Evans was an M.D. (1908) from Johns Hopkins to which he had transferred in 1905 from the University of California School of Medicine. Early in his student days at Hopkins he came under the influence of F. P. Mall and started an active research career mostly related to embryology and the blood vascular system but did no research directly in endocrinology or reproductive physiology. From 1908 until 1915 Evans remained with Mall and spent several summers in Europe where in the laboratory of Edwin Goldman he became fascinated by the use of dyes for vital and supra vital staining. This took him in a new direction, and he began a collaboration with a German chemist Werner Schulemann which culminated in major papers in 1914, published both in English and German. As a young rising star in anatomy with an impressive research record Evans was recruited by President Wheeler to return to the University of California in 1915 as Chairman of its Anatomy Department, and he brought with him many German dyes. Thus was the stage set for the Long-Evans collaboration.

After joining the Zoology Department faculty, Long continued work related to the ovary, and in *Science* in 1916 reported with Quisno "The Ovulation Period of Rats." They thought it was about 11 days, a finding based on the time of appearance of ova in the oviduct after parturition while no male had access to the female. The same year saw Evans' own first paper relating directly to reproductive physiology, and it was concerned with vital staining of the rat's atretic follicle. The following year (1917) the Stockard and Papanicolaou (2) paper on the estrous cycle of the guinea pig was published. This was preceded on August 18 by an authors abstract. It is not possible to reconstruct precisely when the Long-Evans collaboration began but its flowering depended on this 1917 paper. The American Society of Zoologists met in Baltimore in late December 1918, and the Proceedings of that meeting have an abstract of a paper by Long as sole author reporting that the estrous cycle of the rat is "nearly" 5 days. In this was used the new method of timing. There were 10 abstracts, all by Long and Evans, at the American Association of Anatomists Meeting in April 1920. All 10 of these abstracts dealt with the estrous cycle, and the first is rather long and is described as an abstract of a forthcoming monograph. In 1921 an additional 5 abstracts by Long and Evans were published in *The Anatomical Record* plus 4 by Evans and Long which reported attempts to modify the estrous cycle by endocrine means. These latter involved feeding thyroid or removal of the thyroid and feeding anterior lobe of the pituitary or injecting a crude preparation of it intraperitoneally. The only effects seen were in the injected animals in which the cycles stopped or were lengthened but the growth rate increased. This marked the beginning of the long process of isolating and purifying both the gonadotropic hormones and the hypophyseal GH. Aside from the monograph there was no other publication of this work on the estrous cycle although all the abstracts were reprinted as a group in 1969 (3).

The monograph itself consists of 113 pages of text containing 34 tables of data and an additional 3 large tables in the appendix. There are 11 plates with 94 figures consisting of drawings, photomicrographs, as well as colored drawings and paintings. The first three sections make interesting reading in their own right. In addition to an extensive review of what was known about the length of the estrous cycle in many species it tells us the origin of the Long-Evans strain of rats. It was created about 1915 by crossing a wild male Norwegian Grey rat with white females. The wild rat was trapped by Long from the banks of Strawberry Creek as it flowed through the University of California Berkeley campus. The section dealing with the rats used stresses the necessity of animals of full reproductive vigor and careful control of

---

Received August 3, 1991.

"Remembrance" articles discuss people and events as remembered by the author. The opinion(s) expressed are solely those of the writer and do not reflect the view of the Journal or The Endocrine Society.

the animal colony in all respects. There is a section on diet which says a lot about the conditions under which research was done at the time. One is "The colony has been fed with table scraps supplied daily from a large hotel, thus ensuring them with a variety of nutritious food." It goes on to say that the diet for experimental animals was supplemented by whole milk and other substances. Also worth noting is the description of an automatic device for the removal of newborn rats from their mother before they could be nursed, an essential experimental technique. Although not so stated it seems likely that Long himself designed and made this as he did other types of laboratory equipment. He was a master technician and machinist.

After these first few pages the remainder consists of the body of the observational and experimental data plus discussion. First there is a brief account of the gross anatomy of the reproductive tract followed by a detailed description of the estrous cycle and associated changes in all parts of the reproductive tract. This text is abundantly illustrated in the plates which show not only vaginal smears but also histological changes in all reproductive organs. The naming of the stages differs from that used in the lengthy 1920 abstract and have now become stages 1 through 5, with 5 being the diestrous stage. Cornified cells appear in the vaginal smear early in stage 2 and persist into stage 3. Tabular data show the variations in each stage and the overall length of the cycle is based upon many hundreds of observations in 350 adult females. The account of histological changes in the ovary is based upon about 75 animals of which 37 were killed solely with reference to ovulation at precisely timed intervals after the first appearance of cornified cells in the smear, intervals varying from 15 to about 100 h. Ova were present in the oviduct between 18 and 36 h with only two instances of a longer time interval. This is in good agreement with the time ova are found after parturition, the most being between 18 and 26 h. In observations of corpora lutea the vital dyes played an essential part. Table 36 details the staining properties of 83 different vital dyes with respect to their overall staining, distribution in granules of lutein cells, and preservation for histological study. Their use is beautifully illustrated in Color Plate VI which shows 4 paintings of ovaries of rats given Dianil Blue during pregnancy and killed at parturition, and at 4, 9, and 51 days after. The blue ovary at 4 days shows blue corpora of pregnancy and a single set of yellow postovulatory corpora. None of the animals was allowed to nurse, and in succeeding days there were more and more corpora with diminution of the corpora of pregnancy. Two colored microscopic drawings illustrate the different staining properties of old and young lutein cells and one of their conclusions was that a change in the lipid droplets about the end of a normal cycle marked the end of the function of the corpora.

Since the last century it was known there was a postcopulatory vaginal plug, and Long in 1912 had shown that it followed copulation with sterile males (vasectomized) and that ova could be recovered from the oviduct the next day. This led to the demonstration that the length of the following cycle after mating with a sterile male was approximately tripled with persisting corpora lutea, a pseudopregnancy. Exploring the possibility that some "hormonal" component of the ejaculate was causative, preparations of male reproductive tract organs were made. These injected intraperitoneally were ineffective. *In utero* injection of them or of saline, or even failed injections, were effective. This led to finding simple stimulation of the cervix by insertion of a glass rod produced the same pseudopregnancy. Preparations of cervical epithelium were negative, ruling out "hormonal" effects from injury to those cells. After autotransplantation of the ovary in 14 of 19 experiments cycles occurred and insertion of a glass rod into the cervix produced pseudopregnancy, clearly with no direct neural control of ovarian function. Considering the approximate 6-day period between fertilization and implantation they proposed this pseudopregnancy made uterine conditions more optimum for implantation. There remained, however, the unsolved problem of mechanism. The formulation of the concept of neural input to the hypothalamus and this triggering release of releasing factors and hypophyseal hormones was more than a quarter century in the future. In investigating when deciduomata could be produced they found it possible only when cycles were prolonged as in pseudopregnancy or lactation, both associated with persistent functional corpora.

Another group of studies involved transplantation of ovaries with prophetic results. The transplantation of an ovary from an adult rat into a young one did not hasten development of the reproductive tract nor produce cycles. The transplantation of a very immature ovary into a castrated adult female showed immediate growth, ovulation, corpora lutea formation, and the induction of cycles. In neither case did the transplant survive, and the authors realized they were dealing with the problems of tissue incompatibility.

This author was a student of both Long and Evans, and knew the younger of the two on a more than casual basis for almost 40 yr. They had strikingly different personalities and seemed an improbable pair of collaborators. Hopefully this article has made the case each brought their own unique attributes and experiences to their joint arbeit. As one reads the monograph the choice of words and the almost flamboyant style of writing clearly is that of Evans. In the Parkes interview (3) Evans recounts his writing of it and said that when the manuscript was finished he took a copy to Long who was home ill. Long said "I expected that, since you put it all together, you would be the senior author." Evans said "We have to tell the truth occasionally, Dr. Long; this is your work."

Leslie L. Bennett
Professor Emeritus
University of California
San Francisco

References

1. Long JA, Evans HM 1922 The oestrous cycle in the rat and its associated phenomena. Memoirs. University of California, vol 6
2. Stockard CR, Papanicolaou GN 1917 The existence of a typical oestrous cycle in the guinea-pig—with a study of its histological and physiological changes. Am J Anat 22:225–283
3. Parkes AS 1969 Dr. Herbert M. Evans, an interview. J Reprod Fertil 19:1–49

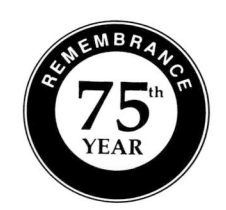

Remembrances of Our Founders: Will Growth Factors, Oncogenes, Cytokines, and Gastrointestinal Hormones Return Us to Our Beginnings?*

Our Founders Had it Right!

The modern concept that hormones regulate both growth and differentiated cell functions was clearly enunciated at the turn of the century by Sir Ernest Starling when he first introduced the term "hormone" during his first Croonian Lecture to the Royal Academy of Physicians on the Chemical Correlation of Body Functions:

"These chemical messengers, however, or 'hormones' (from ορμάω, I excite, or arouse), as we might call them ... (may be divided) into two classes—viz., (1) those which involve increased activity of an organ, or (2) increased growth of a tissue or organ." (1).

Starling's concepts of the endocrine system were extrapolated from his studies of the gastrointestinal hormone secretin and enunciated 9 years before Edward Kendall would isolate thyroxine, 17 years before Banting and Best would isolate insulin, and 21 years before Kendall and Mason would isolate cortisol. It is mind boggling that Starling and his contemporaries were able to envision a global concept of the endocrine system that is remarkably consistent with the new concepts of the endocrine system that are reemerging today. For example, as early as 1891, Brown-Sequard stated, "All the glands-tissues or other organs have special internal secretions which, either by a direct favorable influence, or by preventing the occurrence of noxious reactions, seem to be of great value in maintaining the organism in its normal state" (2). Similarly, in 1895 Professor Edward A. Schafer stated in a lecture to the British Medical Association, "It is not, however, the ductless glands alone which possess the property of (internal secretions), but ... according to our definition, ... apply to any organ of the body" (3). It is thus clear that the founders of endocrinology conceived of chemical mediators as a single system that included, but was not limited to, secretions from the ductless glands.

Redefinition of hormones on the basis of their origin

The emergence of endocrinology as a distinct discipline was not based on the global system of chemical mediation envisioned by our founders but rather on a more restrictive (but more easily defined) model that limited endocrinology to hormones originating in a limited group of strictly defined glands of internal secretion. By the time that The Endocrine Society was founded in 1916 as the Association for the Study of Internal Secretions, most of the gut had been excluded from the endocrine system, along with the brain and most other tissues. The map of the endocrine system shown in Fig. 1 is typical of those that prevailed in standard endocrine textbooks during most of this century.

Consequences of a narrowly defined specialty

The definition of what constitutes a hormone by its source rather than by its function limited our horizons and produced long lasting and serious consequences on the development of our specialty. The pervasive role of chemical mediation in virtually all body processes was poorly integrated into physiological thinking, and when students of my generation wished to learn about endocrinology we could find it all summarized in a single chapter on the ductless glands located in the backs of our textbooks of physiology, biochemistry, or anatomy, along with the special organs of sight, hearing, and smell.

The development of endocrinology as a clinical specialty suffered particularly severe damage by limiting its purview to disorders caused by hypofunction or hyperfunction of a shrinking number of glands. Instead of applying our expertise to the role of chemical mediation in normal physiological processes and common disorders within the mainstream of medical science we allowed endocrinology to become defined in popular thinking as a rather esoteric, if not arcane, discipline. I well remember reading as a medical student the lament by Fuller Albright in *Cecil's Textbook of Medicine* (6) that only fat boys and funny looking patients were referred to endocrinologists, and I was thrilled by his insistence that there was no dividing line between endocrinology and the rest of medicine (6).

Received September 3, 1991.
* This work was supported by NIDDK Grant RO1 AM-1024–35.
"Remembrance" articles discuss people and events as remembered by the author. The opinion(s) expressed are solely those of the writer and do not reflect the view of the Journal of The Endocrine Society.

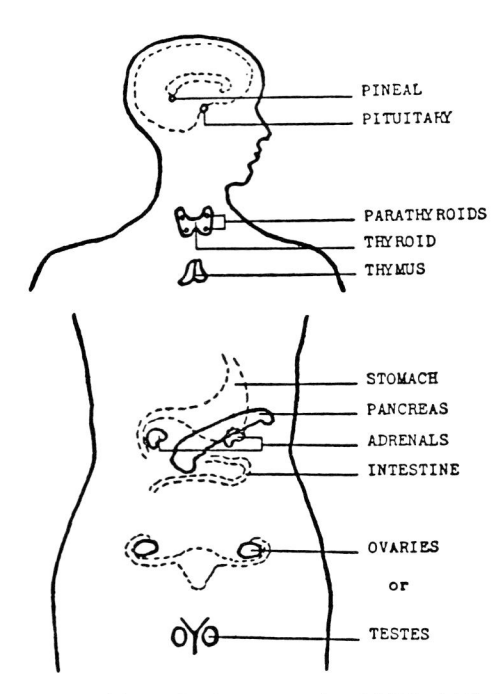

FIG. 1. Diagram of the endocrine system in a 1941 text (4). The legend from a similar drawing in a 1964 text carried the same message: "In (this) figure is shown the location in the human being of the 7 glands which are accepted generally as constituting the endocrine organs—the hypophysis, the thyroid, the parathyroid, the adrenal, the pancreas, the ovary and the testis. The thymus and the pineal are also included, although neither gland has been shown to produce a hormone in the human body." (5).

Endocrinology has prospered in spite of these self-inflicted wounds, and we can take justifiable pride in our accomplishments. We created the technology that made it possible to measure with great precision the concentration of nearly every known hormone in biological fluids, thereby establishing beyond doubt that most physiological and pathological processes are under stringent hormonal control. We have laid down strict criteria for the diagnosis of most endocrine disorders, and we have clearly outlined the principles of effective therapy. Studies of hormone action gave endocrinologists a central role in the exciting new developments in cellular and molecular biology. Our contributions have impacted virtually every discipline in clinical medicine and biomedical science, and our colleagues in other specialties have used the methodology that we developed to integrate one after another of the newly discovered hormones into their own specialties. Such examples include the coopting of erythropoietin and colony-stimulating factors by the hematologists, interleukins and other cytokines by the immunologists, and a myriad of gastrointestinal hormones by the gastroenterologists. This left to endocrinologists only the products of the ductless glands, an anachronism resulting from the archaic definition of our clinical specialty.

The mystique that long surrounded clinical endocrinology is happily beginning to vanish. Commercial reference laboratories now provide easy access to even the most esoteric laboratory procedures, and restrictions have been removed from the prescription of many hormonally active drugs that until recently were available only to investigators. Our accomplishments as teachers have made it possible for graduates of our residencies to diagnose and treat in their local communities most of the endocrine disorders that they formerly referred to academic centers. Such competition from our former students will constitute a threat to our discipline, however, only if we cling to outmoded definitions of the endocrine system and persist in limiting our clinical concerns to the traditional disorders characterized by hypofunction or hyperfunction of the ductless glands.

Recognition that gut hormones, neurotransmitters, and growth factors are indivisible from the rest of the endocrine system

In the recent past, the boundaries of endocrinology have again expanded with our recognition that a single hormone can be produced in multiple tissues, not necessarily including any of the traditional ductless glands. Most if not all of the gastrointestinal hormones, for example, are also formed in brain where they may serve as neurotransmitters. Similarly, cytokines such as the interleukins and tumor necrosis factor(s) have been found in neural tissue where they modulate hypothalamic function and hypophyseal secretion. Such discoveries, along with those of the structure, function, and distribution of POMC and the releasing hormones, have placed endocrinology in the forefront of research on disorders of the nervous system and psychiatric illness.

The discovery of peptide growth factors has opened a similar wealth of new opportunities to those of us whose major concern is the hormonal regulation of growth. One striking difference between peptide growth factors and classical hormones is that growth factors originate in many different sites in the body and appear to act primarily upon neighboring tissues (paracrine effects) or even on their own cells of origin (autocrine effects) rather than on distant tissues that can be accessed only via the blood stream (endocrine effects). These modes of action are not mutually exclusive, however, since a given growth factor may play different roles in different tissues and even function in the classical endocrine manner by transport in the blood to distal target tissues.

Studies of how peptide growth factors fit in with the other systems of humoral regulation assumed a major new dimension with the mounting evidence that they are closely linked with the products of cellular protooncogenes. It is clear that these substances together with growth factors constitute a growth-regulating system that may equal in complexity the entire endocrine system as it was perceived only a few years ago. As regulators of growth and embryonic differentiation these peptides necessarily affect virtually every illness characterized by tissue damage and repair, as well as the processes of aging and neoplastic transformation. This growth-regulating system, however, should not be considered as a separate entity, but rather as a subset of the vast array of chemical mediators that include the cytokines, neurotransmitters, gastrointestinal and hematopoietic hormones, and even the classic hormones originating in the ductless glands.

Where do we go from here?

These new insights on the vast role of chemical mediation in physiology and medicine have created unprecedented opportunities to weave our knowledge and methodologies into the fabric of mainline medicine. To move forward into this new era, however, it will be necessary for us to bring our definition of the endocrine system back into line with the concepts of our founders and convince our colleagues that our expertise and scholarship in the field of chemical mediation is not limited to the hormones produced by the seven or so ductless glands. We might remold long standing and outmoded perceptions of our discipline by changing the names of our endocrine divisions to "Division(s) of Humoral Regulation," although admittedly, not all of us would qualify as humorists.

The problems awaiting our attention are endless and encompass every organ system and every developmental stage from conception to old age. We must venture into the territory of hematologists by asking how their specialized growth factors interact with broad spectrum growth factors and classic hormones in responses to anemia, granulocytopenia, and thrombocytopenia. The techniques of classic endocrinology are particularly well suited for determining what aberrations of the interleukins and other growth factors are at play in congenital and acquired immune deficiency states. We must work with our colleagues in gastroenterology to determine how gut hormones interact with peptide growth factors and other hormones in malnutrition, malabsorption syndromes, and ulcerative disease. Could the atrophic epithelial cells that line the gut of malnourished patients respond to some combination of growth factors and reduce the need for parenteral alimentation? What are the possibilities for accelerating the healing of wounds and burns or for hastening the recovery from injury to liver, kidney, or lungs? Lastly, if neoplastic diseases are fundamentally growth disorders, why should endocrinologists not be at the forefront of cancer research?

The problems awaiting solution by application of the new endocrinology are limited only by our imaginations. The above examples illustrate that the wide range of chemical mediators that are now known plus perhaps an even larger number awaiting discovery are opening new frontiers in every area of physiology and medicine. We need only apply the skills that we have used so successfully in documenting how the traditional hormones function in normal physiology and pathological states. To this end we can begin in our training programs by encouraging new generations of endocrinologists to abandon our traditional insularity and apply our technology to problems that lie outside of traditional endocrine concerns. Our mission has never been stated more clearly than it was by Sir Earnest Starling (7) who in 1905 concluded his famous Croonian Lectures with this passage:

"If, as I am inclined to believe, all of the organs of the body are regulated in their growth and activity by chemical mechanisms similar to those I have described, an extended knowledge of the hormones and their modes of action cannot fail to add largely to the complete control of the body which is the goal of medical science."

Judson J. Van Wyk
Department of Pediatrics
University of North Carolina School
of Medicine

References

1. Starling EH 1905 The Croonian lectures: the chemical correlation of the functions of the body. Lecture 1. Lancet 2:339–341
2. Brown-Séquard CE, D'Arsonval A 1891 Sur les extraits retires des glands et d'autres parties de l'organisme. Archives de Physiologie Normale et Pathologique, Series 5 III:491–506
3. Schafer E 1895 Address in physiology on internal secretions. Lancet 2:321–324
4. Hoskins RG 1941 Endocrinology: the Glands and Their Functions. WW Norton and Co., New York
5. Grollman A 1964 Clinical Endocrinology and its Physiologic Basis. JP Lippincott, Philadelphia
6. Albright F 1944 What is endocrinology? In: Cecil RL (ed) A Textbook of Medicine. WB Saunders, Philadelphia pp 1203–1205
7. Starling EH 1905 The Croonian lectures on the chemical correlation of the functions of the body. Lecture 4. Lancet 2:579–583

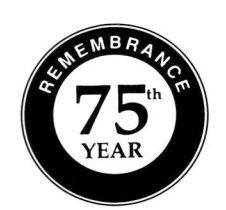

Alfred E. Mirsky and the Foundations of Molecular Biology and Neuroendocrinology

In the 1960s, Alfred Mirsky, Professor at Rockefeller University, was our Ph.D. thesis advisor and helped each of us to lay the foundations of our life's work in neuroendocrinology. Alfred, a pioneer in the field now known as molecular biology, began his research career with his Ph.D. degree in 1926 from the University of Cambridge, Kings College, under the direction of the physiologist Joseph Barcroft. His Ph.D. thesis provided the first demonstration of the reversible denaturation of a protein by demonstrating that heme could be removed from hemoglobin by acetone extraction and that active hemoglobin could be reconstituted by adding back the heme. Alfred's interest in protein denaturation led him in 1936 to Cal Tech to work for a year with Linus Pauling on a hypothesis of protein folding and stabilization by hydrogen bonds.

During the decades before we knew him, Alfred had achieved reknown for his studies of proteins and nucleic acids. After his confrontation with Avery in 1947, in which Alfred questioned whether the pneumococcal transforming factor could be DNA or a protein contaminant, Alfred came over to the side of DNA several years later. In his collaborative studies with Hans Ris, Alfred provided some of the evidence for DNA as hereditary material by showing that diploid cells have a constant DNA content, whereas haploid cells have half as much DNA. Then, with Ris and also Arthur Pollister at Columbia, Alfred began pioneering investigations of chromatin and was the first to note that the content of nonhistone chromosomal proteins is positively correlated with the overall genomic activity of cells. These proteins are now recognized to include sequence-specific regulators of genomic function.

In the 1950s, Alfred pursued his interest in proteins and began to investigate their biosynthesis in cells. Alfred was joined by Marie M. Daly and Vincent G. Allfrey to provide some of the early evidence for the participation of RNA in the formation of proteins by the microsome fraction of cells. Later, with Allfrey, Virginia Littau, and Carolyn J. Burdick, Alfred showed that type H1 histone has a special function of linking together chromosome strands. Allfrey subsequently went on to conduct his own pioneering studies of the past 20 years on the role of histones and their acetylation in the opening of nucleosomes, which occurs during the activation of gene transcription.

When we joined Alfred's laboratory in the 1960s (B. S. McEwen in 1960–1964 and C. Finch in 1965–1969), he was then a very senior figure in the presumptive field of eukaryotic molecular biology and a member of the National Academy of Sciences, presiding over an exciting research group which included Allfrey as well as Eric Davidson, who had come to Rockefeller as a graduate student. Nucleoprotein chemistry and developmental biology were major laboratory themes, and Alfred, who read voraciously and widely, had become fascinated by examples in the biological world of what he called "variable, environmental control of gene expression," *i.e.* how the same hereditary material in all cells can give rise to the differentiated organism and remain involved through the life span in responses to environmental change. Hormones were among his favorite subjects. Many laboratory discussions were triggered by the discoveries in the 1960s of ecdysone effects in insects on the puffing of polytene chromosomes and of vertebrate steroid receptor proteins which locate in the nucleus and bind to DNA. Steroid receptors became for Alfred prime examples of putative protein gene regulators of the nonhistone nucleoprotein class. During this time in the Mirsky laboratory, Eric Davidson had begun work on cytoplasmic factors that regulate gene activity during early development; his article for *Scientific American* (1965) on hormones and gene activity represents another outgrowth from the far-reaching laboratory discussions.

The nervous system was also a favorite topic for Alfred, and he became interested not only in the hormonal control of behavior and neuroendocrine function but also how and why twins are similar in many respect and different in others. His interests in the interactions between heredity and environment also translated into concerns about the social implications of eugenics and views of other scientists about racial differences.

Such was the rich intellectual environment in which we conducted our Ph.D. thesis research. Alfred often expounded upon the findings of Geoffrey Harris on the

---

Received August 27, 1991.

"Remembrance" articles discuss people and events as remembered by the authors. The opinion(s) expressed are solely those of the writers and do not reflect the view of the Journal or The Endocrine Society.

hypothalamo-hypophysial portal blood system and of Emil Witschi, Vera Dantchikoff, Harris, and others on the developmental and endocrine basis of physiological sex differences and the existence of organizing influences (an old term in embryology) at the level of the hypothalamus during a critical phase of development. Alfred viewed these as examples of differential gene expression through hormonal influences. Although very little was known then about the steroid receptors in the brain, Alfred was aware of Donald Pfaff's Ph.D. thesis work at MIT (1966) showing the presence in brain of steroid binding sites and also pointing to the existence of sex differences in hypothalamic neuronal nucleolar size. Through his extensive reading and knowledge in a wide range of areas, Alfred brought the point home to both of us that undoubtedly gene expression was differentially regulated in the brain as a result of developmental influences and was very likely altered during the course of adult life by the hormonal environment. Alfred was aware of the work of Swanson and van der Werff ten Bosch in 1964, which showed that submasculinizing doses of androgens cause a delayed suppression of ovulation that might be a model for accelerated aging. At that time, a few phenomena of aging involving steroid hormones and neuroendocrine function were already indicated: the Pacific salmon that die at first spawning with high stress cortisol levels, and the postmenopausal hot flushes.

We remember how Alfred's refined voice would call out across the laboratory about some article that caught his eye, "Say... have you seen this? It's most remarkable." There were also the lively discussions at afternoon tea, during which Alfred expounded more fully on his views of the biological world and its relationship to social issues. These conversations went on for each of us and for many other associates over many years, as Alfred's vast curiosity and intellectual energy took him and us deep into what have become the fields of molecular biology and neuroscience. For each of us, these conversations still ring loud and clear and give major inspiration to our ongoing work in neuroendocrinology as well as that of our students, to whom we have tried to pass on some of this enthusiasm and love of scholarship.

For B. S. McEwen, the road after Alfred Mirsky led to adrenal steroid receptors in the brain and the study of brain gonadal steroid receptors and sexual differentiation and sexual behavior. He now occupies space which includes part of the old Mirsky laboratory at Rockefeller University.

C. Finch began his studies on aging under Alfred Mirsky's gaze, completing a thesis in 1969 on stress and liver enzyme regulation that led to subsequent studies on the neuroendocrinology of aging.

Bruce S. McEwen, Ph.D.
Professor and Head
Laboratory of Neuroendocrinology
Rockefeller University
Caleb Finch, Ph.D.
ARCO and William F. Kieschnick
  Professor in the Neurobiology of
  Aging
Andrus Gerontology Center
University of Southern California

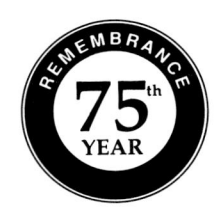

The Early History of the Releasing Factors

The brilliant studies of Harris, in which he showed that intact portal venous connections between the hypothalamus and pituitary gland were essential for normal pituitary function, stimulated a search for the putative neurohumoral agents now termed releasing and inhibiting factors.

The principal problem in the releasing factor field as with all fields in biology was the development of suitable bioassays for the putative neurohormones. A number of abortive attempts were made to establish CRFs by injecting substances into Nembutal-anesthetized rats. These were of little value since the rat responds to many stimuli by a release of ACTH. For example, Martini (1954) injected Pitressin into Nembutal-anesthetized rats and evoked ACTH release, but in view of the vasoactive properties of vasopressin, this could have been attributed to a stress response. Later he applied Pitressin directly to anterior pituitary grafts in the anterior chamber of the eye and obtained ACTH release (1956).

McCann and Brobeck (1954) published the first experiments designed to evaluate ACTH-releasing substances in an animal in which the ubiquitous ACTH release from stress was abolished. McCann (1953) had earlier shown that median eminence lesions would block the ACTH release from stress and the response to epinephrine. Consequently, he ruled out epinephrine as a corticotropin-releasing factor.

McCann and Brobeck showed that a reproducible blockade of the response to stress occurred in animals with severe diabetes insipidus. They used these as assay animals for putative ACTH-releasing substances. In these animals with chronic median eminence lesions, they demonstrated that a high dose of iv Pitressin, a commercially available, partially purified vasopressin, would release ACTH and that this ACTH-releasing action was not shared by oxytocin, the other known neurohypophyseal hormone, or by other putative releasing compounds, such as epinephrine, serotonin, substance P, and histamine. In these animals with chronic lesions, the dose of Pitressin required was very high (5 U), a concentration which we thought would never reach the pituitary via the systemic circulation. It was already known from the work of Verney that stresses of various sorts would release vasopressin and since lesions which produced diabetes insipidus, thereby eliminating vasopressin, were associated with a blockade of ACTH release, we postulated that vasopressin could be the ACTH-releasing hormone via its release into portal vessels and its delivery to the corticotrophs in high concentration.

We later showed (1957) that if we used the animals 48 h after lesions, we had a more sensitive test animal which could respond to as little as 0.1 U iv vasopressin and failed to respond to the abovementioned other putative releasers. Furthermore, synthetic lysine vasopressin kindly donated to us by duVigneaud (Cornell University Medical School, New York, NY) was equally active indicating that the ACTH-releasing activity was caused by vasopressin itself and not a contaminant in Pitressin.

Before that time we had tested acid hypothalamic extracts from beef and rat in the animals with chronic lesions and found them to be inactive. Consequently, we concluded that vasopressin was the ACTH-releasing peptide. Thus, vasopressin was the first releasing factor to be discovered.

Saffran and Schally (1955) developed an *in vitro* system of pituitary incubation and published confirmation of our findings that pressor posterior pituitary preparations caused a release of ACTH, but only from glands which were also incubated in the presence of norepinephrine. In retrospect, it is now apparent why it was necessary to incubate with norepinephrine. It was because of the failure to use preincubation. Therefore, the ACTH released at the time of the initial cutting of the gland presented a very high background, and it was difficult to observe further stimulation. Shortly thereafter in collaboration with B. J. Benfey, Saffran and Schally reported that chromatography of purified vasopressin preparations separated on the chromatogram a zone which released ACTH and yet was devoid of vasopressin. They named this substance CRF. We were unable to confirm this activity by *in vivo* bioassay in our animals with acute hypothalamic lesions.

Independent of Saffran and Schally, Guillemin and Rosenberg (1955) used a hypothalamic-pituitary coculture system to demonstrate increased ACTH release in the presence of hypothalami which could not be accounted for by the small amount of vasopressin released. With Hearn, Guillemin reported that Pitressin would

Received August 27, 1991.
"Remembrance" articles discuss people and events as remembered by the author. The opinion(s) expressed are solely those of the writer and do not reflect the view of the Journal or The Endocrine Society.

release ACTH *in vitro*, but that synthetic vasopressin had no activity. In fact, the response to synthetic vasopressin was only slightly less than that to Pitressin, but not quite statistically significant. Probably if they had increased the dose of synthetic vasopressin slightly, they would have confirmed our *in vivo* results. Because of this finding and the report of Saffran *et al.*, they chromatographed posterior pituitary extracts using a different system than that employed by Saffran *et al.* and reported the separation of fraction D, which ran at the solvent front and contained no pressor activity but would release ACTH *in vitro*. We repeated this work using our *in vivo* assay system and confirmed that fraction D, which was running at the solvent front, was well separated from the pressor portion of the chromatogram ($R_f = 0.4$), which released ACTH in animals with median eminence lesions. Fraction D was ineffective even at a 10-fold higher dose than the pressor fraction from the chromatogram. Guillemin provided us with his fraction D. It produced only a very small response at a dose of 0.5 mg. I elevated the dose to 1 mg, and it was ineffective. These doses were massive compared to the dose of vasopressin required.

At this point, Hearn left Houston for a position at Iowa State, where he worked with a graduate student to purify posterior pituitary extracts. They reported that they could find nothing in such extracts which would release ACTH other than vasopressin. This was also reported later by Porter.

In the meantime, Schally had joined Guillemin in Houston, and they went on to isolate and determine a proposed structure for β-CRF which found its way into biochemistry textbooks for the next 15 years. They also isolated α1 and α2 CRF which were purported to be related to MSH. In his lecture at the Laurentian Hormone Conference in 1963, Guillemin admitted that it was not clear whether there was any meaning to any of the postulated posterior pituitary CRFs. In discussion, Saffran reported that fractionation of 16 batches of posterior pituitary extract had revealed a CRF other than vasopressin only in 6 of the extracts, and he was reporting his CRF in terms of vasopressin units.

The first important work on hypothalamic CRF was performed by Royce and Sayers (1958). They found that stalk median eminence extracts from beef would release ACTH in animals with acute median eminence lesions and went on to purify the active substance. They showed that it was a peptide and obtained preparations which were essentially free from vasopressin. We (1959) showed that even crude median eminence extracts from both rat and beef had CRF activity which could not be accounted for by vasopressin and confirmed the activity of the purified CRF provided to us by Royce and Sayers.

At this point in time, it was quite clear that there were at least two peptides with releasing factor activity, namely, vasopressin and CRF of unknown structure. Another advance was to realize that one could not use the posterior pituitary powders provided by Parke Davis for extraction of releasing factors since, as mentioned above, there was little CRF in posterior pituitaries, and what little was there was masked by the massive amounts of vasopressin, the other CRF.

A number of other people purified hypothalamic CRF, including Porter, Schally, Guillemin, Leeman, and ourselves, but it was not isolated, and its structure was not determined. In retrospect, this failure was probably caused by the large size of the molecule (41 amino acids). Its structure was finally elucidated in 1981 by Vale's group.

Even in these early days (1958), we found that adrenal corticoids probably exerted part of their suppressive action on ACTH release by suppressing the release of vasopressin, since we were able to show that the stress-induced increase in blood vasopressin levels was decreased by treatment of the rats with cortisol. We also demonstrated in collaboration with Yates's group that vasopressin would enhance CRF-induced ACTH release by direct pituitary action in the anesthetized rat (1968), a result confirmed *in vitro* nearly 10 years later by Gillies and Lowry (1978). Furthermore, animals with hereditary diabetes insipidus and complete loss of vasopressin had an impairment in ACTH secretion, albeit relatively small (1966). We postulated that vasopressin and CRF cooperated in control of ACTH release. Studies carried out after the elucidation of the structure of CRF over 20 years later have clearly demonstrated that this is indeed the case.

Nonetheless, neither the role of vasopressin in control of ACTH secretion nor the releasing factor concept was generally accepted in the late 1950s; however, these early experiments led directly to the search for and rapid discovery of the other releasing and inhibiting hormones during the 1960s (see refs. in Ref. 1).

Samuel M. McCann
Department of Physiology
Neuropeptide Division
The University of Texas Southwestern
Medical Center

References

1. McCann SM 1988 Saga of the discovery of hypothalamic releasing and inhibiting hormones. In: McCann SM (ed) People and Ideas in Endocrinology. American Physiological Society, Bethesda, pp 41–62

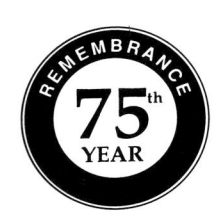

Nettie Karpin Remembers...

I welcome the opportunity to remind the members and the larger scientific world of the many people who have given of their time and energy wholeheartedly to the administration and governance of the Society. This article describes one person who exemplifies all those members whose efforts have brought The Endocrine Society to its present world prominence as a prestigious organization.

I have been fortunate in knowing and working with the eminent scientists of The Endocrine Society during my 14 years of service as the Executive Director of the Society. It has taken much thought to choose one person out of the many who have made distinct and valuable contributions in the administration of The Endocrine Society and in developing it in directions which have served us so magnificently. I would like to introduce you to Alfred E. Wilhelmi, who not only has contributed a great deal to Endocrinology, but also has served this Society in a number of capacities.

Alfred was born in Lakewood, Ohio, is a graduate of Western Reserve University (as it was known in 1933), is a member of Phi Beta Kappa, and a Rhodes Scholar. He received his D.Phil. in Biochemistry from Oxford University in 1937. He was Professor and Chair of Biochemistry at Emory University from 1950 to 1977 and retired in 1979.

Alfred's first acquaintance with the Society came about in 1939, when he began attending meetings with Dr. Jane A. Russell, who became his wife in 1940. Dr. Russell died in 1967, and Alfred lived as a bachelor until he married his present wife, Mary, in 1973. He became a member of the Society in 1960, and he was active until 1989, when he applied for Emeritus status.

During Alfred's years at Emory University, he was known and admired as the "tough Professor." I have just read "A Piece of My Mind" by Joseph E. Hardison, M.D. (JAMA, Feb. 3, 1984, Vol. 251, No. 5). It is titled "Professorial Utterances" and in it I read "Wilhelmi taught us biochemistry. He seemed to know everything about biochemistry. He could not abide ignorance. To answer the question on a test, I had to know the atomic weight of nitrogen. I couldn't remember. We were under the honor system and Dr. Wilhelmi had gone to his laboratory. I entered his lab in a state of fear and trembling. Dr. Wilhelmi always wore the collar of his long, white coat turned up in the back. His eyebrows were bushy and pointed upward in the lateral third. It was very cold in the lab. 'Dr. Wilhelmi, I have forgotten the atomic weight of nitrogen,' I squeaked. He fixed me with gimlet eyes. 'You should have a stake of holly driven through your heart and you should be boiled in oil! The atomic weight of nitrogen is 14'. I answered the question correctly, and I will never forget the atomic weight of nitrogen." Alfred's students never forgot him, we can be sure!

Dr. Wilhelmi was President of the Society, 1968–1969, and as is the way with ex-Presidents, he passed from an active and powerful role to that of an elder statesman. He came to my attention (I had not met him before that time) when President Ernst Knobil asked him to take on the important but extremely unglamorous task of Chair of an *ad hoc* committee on Governance, which had the long and arduous job of rewriting the Society Bylaws. The committee worked long and steadily and came up with revisions that passed overwhelmingly. The other members of this prestigious and hard-working group were Robert M. Blizzard, William T. Ganong, Jack L. Kostyo, Paul L. Munson, and Eugenia Rosemberg.

Alfred had a sustained interest in the Society's publications. He was on the Editorial Board of *Endocrinology* from 1962 to 1974, and he worked with Editor-in-Chief Jack Kostyo 1978–1979, as an Associate Editor. He was appointed to the Publications Committee for two terms, from 1964 to 1970. He worked with the committee as an *ad hoc* member, 1984–1987, and was again appointed a member from 1987–1989, lending his knowledge and interest through two productive years.

Alfred was appointed a member of the Finance Committee for 1976 and 1977, and was Chair of the Committee from 1978 to 1984. His experience on the Publications and Finance Committees coincided with a period when, thanks to the able direction and talent in negotiation of Dr. H. A. Salhanick, Chair of the Publications Committee (1981–1987), the Society's income was sufficient to keep the Journal subscription rates and the Annual Meeting registration fees low enough to encourage members as well as postdocs and students to take advantage of these attractive opportunities. During this period of sizeable income from the Journals, Dr. Wilhelmi, with

---

Received August 19, 1991.

"Remembrance" articles discuss people and events as remembered by the author. The opinion(s) expressed are solely those of the writer and do not reflect the view of the Journal or The Endocrine Society.

Dr. Salhanick's strong support, persuaded Council to establish a Publications Reserve Fund, intended eventually to finance publication of the Journals for a year in case of some unforeseen need. The fund exists today, and it is the backbone, or "Mama's Bank Account," in support of the Society's self-publication of the Journals.

At the risk of boring you, I do want you to recognize the number of Society activities in which Dr. Wilhelmi has been involved, though I won't name them all. He has served on the Awards Committee, the Future Meetings Committee, and the Nominating Committee, to name a few. More recently (1981) Alfred was asked to Chair an *ad hoc* Committee on Archives and History of the Society. This committee functioned intermittently but it did define the requirements for support of the activity.

Finally, all of you have a publication that Alfred wrote in 1988 which describes the Society from its beginnings. It is entitled "The Endocrine Society: Origin, Organization, and Institutions" (*Endocrinology,* **123**:1–43, 1988). I remember how impressed I was with the careful and interesting presentation. A reprint is sent to every Society member and is guaranteed to keep Dr. Wilhelmi in the minds and hearts of us all.

Alfred is now 81 years of age, and is his usual natty, well dressed self. He stands erect, smoothing his beard, and even in retirement, is as interested and knowledgeable as the rest of us. He reads the Journals, attends lectures at Emory, and keeps up with the news in Science. He is present at our Annual Meetings, and is always called upon by friends and colleagues to serve as the memory and history of the years in which he served with great distinction.

I am fortunate to consider him my friend, and as one of the Society members who guided me, listened to me, and provided counsel and solace when things went wrong. He was always ready and available to serve all of our members in the same way.

We wish Alfred Wilhelmi good health and many good years, and we are happy to tell our members about all he has given to us personally and to The Endocrine Society.

Nettie Karpin

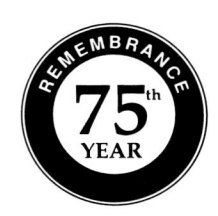

A Failed Assay Opened a New Door in Growth Hormone Research

My initiation to GH took place in the laboratory of Dr. Carl Cori of the Department of Biological Chemistry of the Washington University School of Medicine in 1949. As recounted in an earlier Remembrance by Joseph Larner, a major thrust of that laboratory was to identify the putative inhibitor of hexokinase action, which was postulated to be removed by insulin action. It was known that GH was a potent inhibitor of insulin action in promoting glucose use by muscle, and it was reasoned that GH administration might increase the concentration of this hypothetic inhibitor of hexokinase action. As a naive research fellow fresh from clinical training, I was low man on a research team with Mike Krahl, Rollo Park, and David Brown. Our goal was to characterize GH's action on isolated rat diaphragm. It became soon apparent that the antiinsulin effects observed in this system were not immediate, but required injection of the rats at least 6 h before removal of the diaphragm. In fact, the immediate effect of GH added *in vitro* was an insulin-like stimulation of glucose uptake by the diaphragm. This paradoxical action of GH has never been adequately explained despite its frequent rediscovery over the past 40 yr. This early experience with GH alerted me to the possibility that GH action might require intermediate processes.

Mike Krahl had the idea that the most vigorous and aggressive rats might provide the most potent hexokinase inhibitor. Mixed breed rats were obtained from Anheuser Busch Brewery, who were so fierce that they leapt to attack whenever we approached their cages. As the new boy on the block, I had the privilege of injecting these beer hall bums. I was not sad when these exploratory studies bombed out.

In 1951 I was invited by Dr. Barry Wood, Chairman of the Department of Medicine, to head a new full-time Metabolism Division and establish my own laboratory. Before returning to study of GH, I undertook a collaborative project with Joseph Larner designed to explain the massive inosituria of uncontrolled diabetes mellitus. We found a specific renal tubular inositol reabsorption mechanism, which was inhibited by glucose in rats and human beings.

A second project also turned out well. I had learned from a medical school mentor, S. Howard Armstrong, of the ability of albumin to bind many important small molecules. I was pleased to find that albumin did indeed bind cortisol extensively, but to our surprise the binding of cortisol by serum was much greater than could be attributed to its contained albumin. This observation led to our subsequent investations which established the presence of a corticosteroid binding globulin (transcortin).

While these studies were in progress I was challenged by our inability to evaluate GH secretion in pituitary dwarfism and acromegaly. A few attempts to measure serum GH in hypophysectomiezed rats by measuring the width of the epiphyseal cartilage impressed me with the insensitivity of the method and the tedium of making all the microscopic measurements. With William R. Murphy, I showed that the uptake of ^{35}S-sulfate by cartilage *in vivo* was a very sensitive indicator of the GH status of rats and the defect in sulfation present in hypophysectomized rats could be completely restored within 24 h by treating the rats with GH.

In 1955, I was joined in the laboratory by William D. Salmon, Jr., a physician who had just completed his clinical training. Bill undertook the development of what we hoped would be a superior GH assay. He rapidly established reproducible methods for measuring ^{35}S-sulfate uptake by hypophysectomized rat cartilage *in vitro*. This was the day of small science and Bill performed all the incubations and radioactive measurements himself. β-emitters were detected then in a gas flow counter with planchets individually fed by hand. In addition, Bill had clinical responsibilities in the endocrine consultation service. Such were the iron men of those days. When he added bovine GH to these incubations of hypophysectomized rat cartilage, we were at first very disappointed to find that the stimulation of uptake was only a small fraction of that which we had observed with *in vivo* administration of GH. Having been alerted to the possibility of indirect actions of GH, we next compared the effects of incubation of the hypophysectomized rat costal cartilage segments with diluted normal and hypophysec-

Received September 19, 1991.
"Remembrance" articles discuss people and events as remembered by the author. The opinion(s) expressed are solely those of the writer and do not reflect the view of the Journal or The Endocrine Society.

tomized rat serum. We were delighted to find that the ^{35}S-sulfate uptake in the presence of normal serum was more than 200% greater than that in hypophysectomized rat serum. The addition of GH to hypophysectomized serum did not restore *in vitro* activity, but GH administration *in vivo,* however, did restore the activity *in vitro*. We postulated that the effect of GH was attributable to an inducible "sulfation factor."

In biological research an important, but seldom admitted ingredient, is luck. We had chosen a target tissue which exhibited only a very small response to direct addition of GH, but had a major response to the high levels of sulfation factor (insulin-like growth factor I) present in normal rat serum. In contrast, hypophysectomized rat serum has virtually undetectable concentrations of both insulin-like growth factor I and II. The second ingredient of success in biological research is to recognize when you are lucky and for this we were well prepared.

William H. Daughaday
Irene E. and Michael M. Karl
Professor of Metabolism in Medicine, Emeritus
Washington University School of Medicine

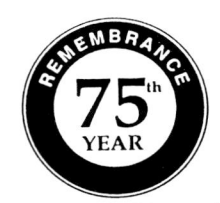

NIH Scientists Develop Specific Assays for Human Chorionic Gonadotropin

The setting

It was early springtime in Bethesda when I arrived in 1969. At 25 yr of age and fresh out of my Ph.D. studies, I couldn't have dreamed of the postdoctoral research and career development opportunities that were about to arrive before me at the NIH. The particular story I am about to tell played a significant role in my formative years as an investigator not only throughout 15 yr at NIH, but even to this day, more than 7 yr after I departed.

Inevitably, history worthy of being told centers on those individuals who played pivotal roles and who also had significant relationships to the persons giving attention to the story. In this case, the senior characters were Roy Hertz, Bill Tullner, Mort Lipsett, and, most especially, Griff Ross: Roy and Bill, because they took a big chance in bringing me into training and taught me so much about bioassays for gonadotropins and sex steroid hormones; Mort, because he encouraged my administrative skills and pointed the way through NIH politics; and Griff, because he showed me how to enjoy the rigors of scientific investigation through the people who become your collaborators and friends for life.

A brief version of the history of this quartet is that Roy Hertz had founded the Endocrinology Branch in NCI in the late 30s. Bill Tullner had joined him in the mid-40s. Mort and Griff were selected to train with Roy in the late 50s. All had remained while rising to leadership roles in NCI. Meantime, the administration of President Kennedy had set forth those policies which, during LBJ's Presidential tenure, resulted in creation of the NICHHD. At the time of my arrival, Roy and Bill had "moved" programmatically into the new Institute, whereas Mort and Griff were still in NCI. By the end of 1970, they too would join us in NICHHD to form the unified Reproduction Research Branch. Several dozen currently prominent endocrinologists in medicine, pediatrics, OB/GYN, and basic reproductive endocrinology trained in this program during the era described herein. Although the remembrances of each of us involved will differ somewhat, I know that a certain familiarity will be recalled by many people active in The Endocrine Society today.

The science

Among the chief contributions of Roy Hertz and his collaborators was the diagnosis and treatment of choriocarcinoma and hydatiform mole, "reproductive cancers" associated with nongestational elevations of hCG. Research and clinical treatment of these diseases in Hertz's lab stretched back more than 20 yr, predating my arrival by several generations of physician/scientist trainees. Although several *in vivo* bioassays and cell culture systems (including the well known BeWo cell line, named for Betty Woods, one of Hertz's long surviving patients) had been used, the mouse uterine weight (MUW) bioassay for hCG in 24-h urinary extracts produced by kaolin-acetone precipitation was the standard test system for monitoring hCG titers in these patients. Among the roles of servitude that befell us as trainees, along with an outstanding technical cadre, was urine collection, processing, mouse injections (a.m. and p.m. for 3 days), and autopsy on day 4 for MUW. Given all the dilutions required to quantitate the patient's urinary hCG titers, we usually tested 500 mice twice per week, including every weekend and holiday, nonstop. That's over 50,000 dissections of the mouse uterus per annum! Then, of course, we had our research to do as well.

Many of you will recall that RIA came into prominence worldwide in the decade of the 1970s. Two of the earliest pioneers of RIAs for gonadotropins were Bill Odell and Griff Ross, along with their several collaborators (1). Among their better anti-hCG sera was B-1 (bunny one—simple things work best in the government). The B-1 RIA was a terrific advance because it manifested a high degree of cross-reactivity with both hCG and hLH (also useful for some nonhuman primates, see below); thus, studies of the menstrual cycle, pregnancy and hCG-producing neoplasia were all enabled simultaneously (2). Well, we were all quite eager to use RIA to monitor hCG titers and to get away from the time, expense, and drudgery of 50,000 plus mouse autopsies every year. Trouble was, we couldn't use the new B-1 RIA alone for patients receiving chemotherapy and/or surgical treatment because low levels of hLH and/or hCG cross-

---

Received October 21, 1991.

"Remembrance" articles discuss people and events as remembered by the author. The opinion(s) expressed are solely those of the writer and do not reflect the view of the Journal or The Endocrine Society.

reacted without sufficient specificity. While this was also true for the MUW bioassay, we had almost 20 yr of background data in patients on which to judge the interpretation of MUW results. Then too, the RIA might have given us spurious data, because it didn't necessarily indicate the biologically active moieties of hCG (or hLH). A second problem was that the amount of B-1 antiserum of good titer was limiting, thereby precluding its dissemination to others on a broad scale.

Enter Judy Vaitukaitis and Glenn Braunstein, who with Griff made the now famous SB6 antiserum, leading to the first widely available and well characterized βhCG RIA, having markedly improved specificity for hCG over hLH (3). But wait; this part of the story derives from Columbia P & S and the laboratory of Bob Canfield with his able co-workers Frank Morgan and Steve Birken. Together, they purified hCG, dissociated its subunits, and sent purified fractions to Griff for quantitative biological activity determinations (4–7). This advance was ultimately an outgrowth from the molecular characterization and amino acid sequencing studies spanning an era when Darryl Ward, Leo Reichert, and Harold Papkoff were teaching us the structures and amino acid sequences of LH and FSH as well. I recall that Rees Midgley and Al Parlow were among the many major contributors to these advances. Learning that the α-subunits were highly conserved among hypophyseal peptides and that the β-subunits conferred functional specificity to these peptide hormones, revealed one of nature's best secrets in endocrinology to that time (8–10). Let us recall, too, that this progress on hCG isolation and purification was accelerated by the farsighted research contract support provided by the Contraceptive Development Branch, NICHHD (Gabe Bialy) from 1969 through the next decade.

Although the βhCG RIAs brought a striking improvement in specificity, patients having very low to nil hCG titers were difficult to separate from those excreting detectable levels of hLH (11). Soon, we set forth to make an ultra-specific hCG assay based on the unique carboxyl terminal peptide (CTP) sequence of the hCG β-subunit. Stepwise peptide synthesis by Shuji Matsuura and Harry Chen led us to identify the principal antigenic sites in the CTP region of 28 amino acids. From there, we made antisera to these peptide fragments, the first good one being H-93. Along the way, we encountered another surprise, that the urine of normal nonpregnant, nonneoplastic persons contained an hCG-like entity (not hLH) that cross-reacted with even the most specific hCG assays and expressed typical biological activity in Maria Dufau's rat interstitial cell *in vitro* bioassay (12–16). Thanks to Mother Superior Mary Catherine and her group of cooperative nuns at the Sister's of Mercy retirement home in Potomac, MD, I was able to obtain large quantities of postmenopausal women's urine, as well as samples from children with Klinefelter's Syndrome. We found that in these states of hypergonadotropin secretion more of the hCG-like material was excreted than from people with functioning gonadal feedback. About the same time Glen Braunstein reported an hCG-like factor in human testis tissue (17); also Bill Odell showed this material is nonendocrine tissues (18). Collectively, we reasoned that the explanation was "gene leakage"—that the promotor might not absolutely shut-off the nucleotide region(s) responsible for hCG production.

These advances sparked rapid progress in the comparative study of chorionic and pituitary gonadotropins of many primate species, including apes, baboons, macaques, and new world monkeys (19–33). Frequently, we worked in cooperation with Bill Peckam in Ernie Knobil's laboratory of the University of Pittsburgh. Ultimately, primate RIA reagents for CG, LH, and FSH were made available for worldwide dissemination through the Hormone Distribution Officer. A special achievement was development of the NIH Non-Human Primate Urinary Pregnancy Test Kit (based on H-26 antiserum against oLHβ) which was supplied gratis worldwide to more than 3000 reproductive biologists, teratologists, zoologists, primate breeders, and other investigators from 1973 through 1986. Again, Gabe Bialy had shown the uncommon wisdom to invest in the potential of others and thereby amplify their productivity beyond expectations.

The significance

In terms of scientific significance, I believe that the work cited has revealed its own value over the 15 to 20 intervening years, both to basic studies in endocrinology and to applied indications in the clinical management of patients today. However, I hope this history conveys some additional significance to older and younger endocrinologists alike: 1) that the best recipe for mentoring young physicians and scientists is to create and sustain a milieu of open and free collaboration with investigators having conjoining skills, with emphasis on generosity and sharing of results and recognition; 2) that basic research and clinical advances really are linked in an ever repeating spiral of knowledge and understanding; and 3) that qualifications for research funding that require knowing the end-product before the support is given, restricts and curtails the very genius inherent to enthusiastic pursuit of scientific inquiry.

My last point relates to the transient nature of an optimal research environment. It's a tenuous, precious, and fragile ecology, seldom enduring for more than a few years in any program. By 1976, Griff and Mort had moved on to direct the activities of the NIH Clinical Center. The once huge Reproduction Research Branch was divided tripartite, with new leadership from Kevin Catt, Lynn Loriaux (Developmental Endocrinology Branch), and myself (Pregnancy Research Branch). For all of those whose careers passed through this story ahead of me, concurrently or since, or those who have experienced similar courses elsewhere, this is my version of the NIH era when specific assays for hCG were developed.

Gary D. Hodgen, Ph.D.
Professor and President
The Jones Institute for Reproductive Medicine
Department of Obstetrics and Gynecology
Eastern Virginia Medical School

References

1. Odell WD, Ross GT, Rayford PL 1967 Radioimmunoassay for luteinizing hormone in human plasma or serum physiological studies. J Clin Invest 46:248–255
2. Marshall JR, Hammond CB, Ross GT, Jacobson A, Rayford P, Odell WD 1968 Plasma and urinary chorionic gonadotropin during early human pregnancy. Obstet Gynecol 32:760–764
3. Viatukaitis JL, Braunstein GD, Ross GT 1972 A radioimmunoassay which specifically measures human chorionic gonadotropin in the presence of human luteinizing hormone. Am J Obstet Gynecol 113:751–758
4. Morgan FJ, Canfield RE 1971 Nature of the subunits of human chorionic gonadotropin. Endocrinology 88:1045–1053–1055
5. Morgan FJ, Birken S, Canfield RE 1973 Letter: human chorionic gonadotropin: a proposal for the amino acid sequence. Mol Cell Biochem 2:97–99
6. Morgan FJ, Birken S, Canfield RE 1975 Amino acid sequence of human chorionic gonadotropin. J Biol Chem 250:5247–5258
7. Morgan FJ, Canfield RE, Vaitukaitis JL, Ross GT 1974 Properties of the subunits of human chorionic gonadotropin. Endocrinology 94:1601–1606
8. Vaitukaitis JL, Ross GT, Reichert LE Jr, Ward DN 1972 Immunologic basis for within and between species cross-reactivity of luteinizing hormone. Endocrinology 91:1337
9. Louvet JP, Harman SM, Nisula BC, Ross GT, Birken S, Canfield R 1976 Follicle-stimulating activity of human chorionic gonadotropin: effect of dissociation and recombination of subunits. Endocrinology 99:1126
10. Louvet J-P, Ross GT, Birken S, Canfield RE 1974 Absence of neutralizing effect of antisera to the unique structural region of human chorionic gonadotropin. J Clin Endocrinol Metab 39:1155–1158
11. Schreiber JR, Rebar RW, Chen HC, Hodgen GD, Ross GT 1976 Limitation of the specific radioimmunoassay for hCG in the management of trophoblastic neoplasms. Am J Obstet Gynecol 125:705–707
12. Chen HC, Hodgen GD, Matsuura S, Lin LJ, Gross E, Reichert LE Jr, Birken S, Canfield RE, Ross GT 1976 Evidence for a gonadotropin from non-pregnancy subjects that has physical, immunological, and biological similarities to human chorionic gonadotropin. Proc Natl Acad Sci 73:2885–2889
13. Hodgen GD, Chen HC, Dufau ML, Klein TA, Mishell DR 1978 Transitory hCG-like activity in the urine of some IUD users. J Clin Endocrinol Metab 46:689–701
14. Ayala AR, Nisula BC, Chen HC, Hodgen GD, Ross GT 1978 Highly sensitive radioimmunoassay for chorionic gonadotropin in human urine. J Clin Endocrinol Metab 47:767–773
15. Matsuura S, Ohashi M, Chen HC, Hodgen GD 1979 A human chorionic gonadotropin-specific antiserum against synthetic peptide analogs to the carboxyl-terminal peptide of its β-subunit. Endocrinology 104:396–401
16. Ohashi M, Matsuura S, Chen HC, Hodgen GD 1980 Comparison of in vivo and in vitro neutralization of human chorionic gonadotropin (hCG) activities by antisera to hCG and a carboxyl-terminal fragment of the β-subunit. Endocrinology 107:2034–2040
17. Braunstein GD, Rasor J, Wade ME 1975 Presence in normal human testes of chorionic gonadotropin-like substance distinct from human luteinizing hormone. N Engl J Med 293:1339
18. Yoshimoto Y, Wolfsen AR, Odell WD 1977 Human chorionic gonadotropin-like substance in non-endocrine tissues of normal subjects. Science 197:575
19. Nixon WE, Hodgen GD, Niemann WH, Ross GT, Tullner WW 1972 Urinary chorionic gonadotropin in middle and late pregnancy in the chimpanzee. Endocrinology 90:1105–1109
20. Hodgen GD, Nixon WE, Vaitukaitis JL, Tullner WW, Ross GT 1973 Neutralization of primate chorionic gonadotropin activities by antisera against the subunits of human chorionic gonadotropin in radioimmunoassay and bioassay. Endocrinology 92:705
21. Hodgen GD, Ross GT 1974 Pregnancy diagnosis by a hemagglutination inhibition test for urinary macaque chorionic gonadotropin (mCG). J Clin Endocrinol Metab 38:927–930
22. Hodgen GD, Tullner WW, Vaitukaitis JL, Ward DN, Ross GT 1974 Specific radioimmunoassay of chorionic gonadotropin during implantation in rhesus monkeys. J Clin Endocrinol Metab 39:457–464
23. Hodgen GD, Niemann WH 1975 Application of the subhuman primate pregnancy test kit to pregnancy diagnosis in baboons. Lab Anim Sci 25:757–759
24. Hodgen GD, Wolfe LG, Ogden JD, Adams MR, Descalzi CC, Hildebrand DF 1976 Diagnosis of pregnancy in marmosets: hemagglutination inhibition test and radioimmunoassay for urinary chorionic gonadotropin. Lab Anim Sci 26:224–229
25. Hodgen GD, Niemann WH, Turner CK, Chenk HE 1976 Diagnosis of pregnancy in chimpanzees using the nonhuman primate pregnancy test kit. J Med Primatol 5:247–252
26. Hodgen GD, Wilks JW, Vaitukaitis JL, Chen HC, Papkoff H, Ross GT 1976 A new radioimmunoassay for follicle-stimulating hormone in macaques: ovulatory menstrual cycles. Endocrinology 99:137–145
27. Chen HC, Hodgen GD 1976 Primate chorionic gonadotropins: antigenic similarities to the unique carboxyl-terminal peptide of hCGb subunit. J Clin Endocrinol Metab 43:1414–1417
28. Hodgen GD, Turner CK, Smith EE Bush RM 1977 Pregnancy diagnosis in the orangutan (Pongo pygmaeus) using the subhuman primate pregnancy test kit. Lab Anim Sci 27:99–101
29. Nixon WE, Chen HC, Hodgen GD 1977 Antigenic similarities to HCG subunits among chorionic gonadotropins of nonhuman primates. J Med Primatol 6:195–202
30. Hodgen GD, Stolzenberg SJ, Jones DCL, Hildebrand DF, Turner CK 1978 Pregnancy diagnosis in squirrel monkeys: hemagglutination test, radioimmunoassay, and bioassay of chorionic gonadotropin. J Med Primatol 7:59–64
31. Kleiman DG, Gracey DW, Hodgen GD 1978 Urinary chorionic gonadotropin levels in pregnant golden lion tamarins: preliminary observations. J Med Primatol 7:333–338
32. Hall RD, Hodgen GD 1979 Pregnancy diagnosis in owl monkeys (*Aotus trivigatus*): evaluation of the hemagglutination inhibition test for urinary chorionic gonadotropin. Lab Anim Sci 29:345–348
33. Stolzenberg SJ, Jones DCL, Barth RA, Hodgen GD, Madan SM 1979 Studies with timed-pregnant squirrel monkeys (*Saimiri sciureus*). J Med Primatol 8:29–38

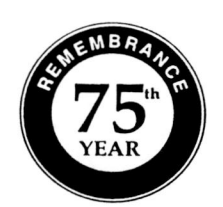

Reminiscences of the Twelfth Floor of the Clinical Center of NIH (circa 1965)

During medical school I became fascinated with endocrinology and determined to have a career in endocrine research. After finishing school in 1963, I decided that the best place to combine research with the mandatory service obligation was the National Institutes of Health. I remember going for my interviews with the chiefs or interviewers from the various laboratories and branches at the NIH that year. Most of the people with whom I visited were cordial and listened politely as I explained that I had not really done much research, but that I planned to spend the subsequent year in a special fellowship program. However, the inescapable fact remained that there was no bibliography attached to my application.

My last meeting of the day was with a member of the Endocrinology Branch of the National Cancer Institute, a branch that occupied parts of the 12th and 10th floors of the Clinical Center. This interview was different. Instead of seeing me in his office, Griff Ross interviewed me while peering into a microscope looking for melanin granule dispersion in the toe webs of live frogs. Griff, who later shared a microscopically small office with me for several years, had a knack for putting people at ease. He related much about his own career, which included returning from general practice to do special training with Dr. Al Albert at the Mayo Clinic. Fortunately, Griff put a great deal of emphasis on motivation, and I was selected as one of the Clinical Associates for the next incoming group. On returning to Duke, I found that one of my fellow interns, Bert O'Malley, had also been selected to be in the same group.

When we arrived in Bethesda in 1965, we found a remarkably talented group of scientists in our group. Branch Chief Roy Hertz was in the process of retiring. Mortimer Lipsett was becoming the new Chief, and Griff Ross the Associate Chief.

These two men complemented each other almost perfectly, and ultimately ended up as the Director and Associate Director of the Clinical Center, many years later. Their talents formed an impressive blend for the neophyte investigator. Mort was or bordered on brilliance. He was extraordinarily decisive, and while he was usually patient, he did not suffer fools gladly. We learned to read Mort's reactions quickly to see if we were on the right track with a research plan. While Mort was brilliant and extremely athletic, he was not always graceful in the laboratory. On one occasion, he knocked a laboriously developed steroid extraction on the floor and was seen trying to pipette the puddled remainder off the tile. Hildegard Wilson, entering the room at this inopportune time, wheeled about and started out of the room, saying over her shoulder "I will pretend I never saw this!"

Mort's greatest research strength was his penetrating intellect. Griff, on the other hand, possessed a phenomenal memory and an amazing sense of humor. He usually had an East Texas expression for any occasion. An example might be, "He wouldn't cross the road to see a chigger eat an elephant," or when an experiment failed, "you can't get all the roses to bloom in May." While Griff had excellent judgment and could provide compelling arguments for a particular course of action, he often deferred final decisions to Mort. Griff also was a natural entertainer, had an impressive repertoire of songs, and played a bagful of harmonicas. Many social occasions ended with Griff holding forth on the harmonica. In fact, Griff would play so vigorously that at times we worried about his cardiovascular system.

Perhaps one of the most remarkable aspects of the Branch was the other people in this relatively small group that began in the NCI and later transferred to NICHD. The group was quite collegial with social gatherings at Chinese restaurants and along the old Georgetown Canal. Among the group were three future Presidents of The Endocrine Society and numerous nascent scientists. On my arrival, in addition to Mort Lipsett and Griff Ross, the senior staff was made up of William Odell and Stan Korenman. Bob Utiger had just left after collaborating with Bill Odell and Jack Wilber on the TSH RIA. Kevin Catt and Maria Dufau joined later, and Marvin Kirschner was on sabbatical. It is impossible to mention everyone. Bill Tullner was in charge of many of the animal activities until he recruited Gary Hodgen to work with him. The Clinical Associates included Chuck Hammond, Wayne Bardin, Bert O'Malley, Howard Kulin, Arlene

---

Received October 21, 1991.
"Remembrance" articles discuss people and events as remembered by the author. The opinion(s) expressed are solely those of the writer and do not reflect the view of the Journal or The Endocrine Society.

Rifkind, and myself. Over the next few years new staff and Fellows included Bill McGuire, David Rodbard, Judy Vaitukaitus, Itamar Abrass, Geoff Rosenfield, Wylie Hembree, George Schneider, Lynn Loriaux, Glenn Braunstein, Bruce Nisula, Ira Pastan, Harold Varmus, Tony Means and numerous others who have gone on to distinguished careers. A few like Loriaux, Rodbard, and Nisula stayed for 20 yr or more.

There were several memorable events in the program. Hertz and Li had been the first to treat and cure choriocarcinoma with chemotherapy. When I first arrived, there were still a large number of choriocarcinoma patients being treated. These patients were monitored by the mouse uterine weight bioassay. Each Wednesday at our conference Griff Ross would bring in the book of bioassays, the "Good Book" as he called it, to design the treatments for the week ahead. As the RIAs for LH and hCG began to be developed, they were also measured; but the bioassay remained the mainstay of treatment for many years.

Both Mort and Griff were excellent clinicians as were many others in the group. Griff particularly liked to demonstrate physical findings. He had a group of approximately 50 patients with Turner's Syndrome. He always liked to comment on their short stature. Arlene Rifkind was petite to diminutive at an even 5 feet. Griff delighted in asking Arlene to stand back to back with the Turner's patients to show how short they were. Arlene was gracious about this even when quite pregnant.

We always seemed to be surrounded by urine collection bottles. Shortly after arriving in Bethesda, O'Malley decided to do a steroid study using monkey urine. Either the preservative was bad or the process flawed, so that the stench of old monkey urine permeated the 12th floor for what seemed like weeks. Howard Kulin and Arlene Rifkind were trying to work out gonadotropin secretion in children and had gallons of urine stashed in all available refrigerated spaces.

One of my strongest memories is of Bert O'Malley's chicken studies. Stan Korenman had started a project to look at the chick oviduct after estrogen stimulation. Bert had decided to work with Stan on this project, but Stan and my mentor, Bill Odell, left for Harbor General Hospital in California at the end of our first year. Bert picked up the oviduct project with very little help other than a superb technician. However, in order to carry out the experiments, large numbers of chicks had to be injected every 6 h around the clock for 6 successive days. Bert dutifully came in every 6 h to make the evening, night, and holiday injections. I always believed Bert deserved every accolade after watching him try to reach recalcitrant chickens hiding in the far corners of a side-entry cage in the wee hours of the morning.

One other happy outcome of the Branch activities was the enthusiasm for personal advancement. The Chief Technician in the Branch was Phil Rayford. He was obviously extremely intelligent, able to get every technique to work, and was invaluable to Bill Odell and Griff Ross in the development of the RIAs for LH and FSH. He was able to go to the University of Maryland while still working at the NIH and get his Ph.D. in Reproductive Physiology. Phil subsequently became Vice Chair of the Surgery Department in Galveston and currently is Chair of Physiology at the University of Arkansas Medical Center.

The scientists on the 12th and 10th floors in the Endocrinology Branch were unique individuals in happy equilibrium with a particularly stimulating research environment. Those were the halcyon days.

Peter O. Kohler, M.D.
Oregon Health Sciences University

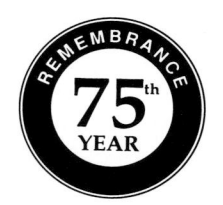

Remembrance of an Unexpected Turn in the Road*

Readers of this article will all remember the times when everything conceivable was going wrong in the laboratory. I recall such a situation some 20 yr ago, and I am writing this article to remind my colleagues that this does not necessarily presage disaster but may in fact be the harbinger of better things to come. In our case, what appeared at first blush to be a set of uninterpretable results led to the recognition of the nuclear receptor for T_3. Our laboratory at the time was located at the Montefiore Hospital and Medical Center in the Bronx, NY and my colleagues in this series of studies were Drs. Diona Koerner, Harold Schwartz, and Martin Surks.

The principal interests of the laboratory were related to the kinetics of distribution and metabolism of thyroid hormone, especially insofar as these parameters were influenced by plasma and tissue binding of T_4 and T_3. We had observed a rapid exchange of T_4 and T_3 between plasma and cellular pools and hypothesized that the partition between them was determined by the balance of cellular and plasma protein binding.

As part of this effort, Dr. Schadlow, a postdoctoral endocrine fellow in our laboratory, undertook the study of the kinetics of exchange of T_4 and T_3 between plasma and selected tissues of the rat, including liver, kidney, pituitary, and brain. For this purpose [^{131}I]T_4 or [^{131}I]T_3 was injected iv, animals killed at timed intervals, blood and organs removed, and the ratio of radioactive hormone content in the tissue and plasma content determined. Dr. Schadlow encountered no problem in defining these ratios for liver, kidney, and brain for both hormones and in determining the pituitary/plasma ratio for T_4. However, he ran into unexpected difficulty in obtaining consistent results for the steady state pituitary/plasma T_3 ratio. His results seemed totally erratic and our research in this area came to a sudden stop.

Before abandoning these efforts altogether, however, we took another look at the data. We noted that the pituitary/plasma T_3 ratio appeared to fall systematically in successive experiments carried out with the same shipment of radioactive T_3. At the time ^{131}I was the only radioactive nuclide of iodine commercially available for labeling iodothyronines. The radiolabeled T_3 thus decayed with a half time of only 8.1 days instead of the 60 days which is characteristic of ^{125}I-labeled iodothyronines currently available. The earlier preparations were also of low specific activity compared to current standards. As time elapsed following the receipt of a shipment of ^{131}I-labeled T_3 Dr. Schadlow used progressively larger volumes of the preparation to maintain approximately the same counting rate in his biological samples. This maneuver added substantially to the mass of T_3 injected. It occurred to us that the progressive fall in the pituitary plasma ratio could reflect stereospecific binding sites for T_3 in the pituitary, sites which could be readily saturated by increasing the mass of injected T_3. We verified this hypothesis by analyzing the effects on the tissue/plasma ratio of a dose of tracer T_3 and T_4 supplemented with progressively increasing amounts of the cold hormone. The presence of limited capacity sites in the pituitary for T_3 but not T_4 was reported in the June 16, 1972 issue of *Science* (1). The concept that these sites might mediate hormone action appeared attractive in the context of concurrent developments which indicated that T_4 is converted to the biologically more active hormone T_3 (2).

We wondered, however, why we had been unable to demonstrate such receptors in liver or kidney. Subcellular fractionation studies in animals injected with tracer levels of T_3 and graded dose of the corresponding unlabeled iodothyronine showed that both liver and kidney did possess specific binding sites in the nuclei of these tissues. However, such specifically bound to T_3 represented only about 15% of the radioactive tracer T_3 in the cell as a whole. This fraction would not be readily detectable in unfractionated liver and kidney. Even though based entirely on observations in experimental animals, our report was published as a *Rapid Communication* in the August 12, 1972 issue of *The Journal of Clinical Endocrinology and Metabolism* (3). *Endocrinology* did not carry *Rapid Communications* at that time. By mutual agreement between the two journals, *Rapid Communications*, regardless of the species under study, were handled by *JCEM*. A subsequent report (4) showed that fully 50% of total T_3 contained in the anterior pituitary is specifically bound to the nuclear sites. This provided an explanation for our ability to demonstrate specific binding sites in unfractionated pituitary.

The observation of specific nuclear binding sites was

Received October 14, 1991.

"Remembrance" articles discuss people and events as remembered by the author. The opinion(s) expressed are solely those of the writer and do not reflect the view of the Journal or The Endocrine Society.

* Supported by NIH Grant DK-19812.

rapidly confirmed and extended by our colleagues (5, 6). The contribution of Samuels and his associates were particularly important inasmuch as they demonstrated that similar nuclear receptors in rat pituitary cell lines transduced the effect of thyroid hormone in regulating GH gene expression. Studies in several laboratories including our own showed that nuclear sites were nonhistone chromatin proteins. Methods were developed to allow the quantitation of the receptors in whole nuclei and nuclear extracts. Evidence that these sites were true receptors involved in the initiation of thyroid hormone action was soon forthcoming from a comparison of biological activity and nuclear occupancy as well as the correlation of thyromimetic effects of T_3 hormone analog with their affinity to nuclear sites.

The concept that the nucleus was involved in the initiation of thyroid hormone action was not novel, having been first advanced in a series of prescient studies by Tata and Widnell in the mid 1960s (7). Their concepts, however, were not universally accepted. Competing hypotheses had been advanced to suggest that thyroid hormones exerted a direct effect on the mitochondrial and microsomal fractions (8). Even Tata himself eventually adopted the eclectic viewpoint that thyroid hormones have multiple subcellular sites of initiation (9). The demonstration of a specific site of interaction of T_3 and DNA-associated receptor, however, resulted in increasing support of the nuclear hypothesis. More recently the recognition that the genes coding for the T_3 receptors are part of a superfamily of genes coding for the steroid, vitamin D, and retinoic acid receptors has further stimulated interest in the area and has revealed an unexpected diversity in the structure of the thyroid hormone receptor.

Our story emphasizes the role of sheer luck in the discovery process. Had Dr. Schadlow omitted the pituitary from the tissues under investigation no discrepancies would have been observed. Had ^{125}I with its much longer half-life been available, no problems would have arisen. Clearly, the precedence of nuclear receptors for steroid hormones, the earlier studies of Tata, and the recognition of the importance of T_4 to T_3 conversion were all important factors in helping us to identify nuclear T_3 receptors. Progress is never made in a vacuum.

Perhaps the reader can take comfort from our experience the next time that he or she encounters inconsistent laboratory results. My advice to the investigator would be to "hang in," and take another look at the data.

Jack H. Oppenheimer
Section of Endocrinology and Metabolism
Department of Medicine
University of Minnesota

References

1. Schadlow A, Surks M, Schwartz H, Oppenheimer J 1972 Specific triiodothyronine binding sites in the anterior pituitary of the rat. Science 176:1252–1254
2. Braverman LE, Ingbar SH, Sterling K 1970 Conversion of thyroxine to triiodothyronine in athyreotic human subjects. J Clin Invest 49:855–864
3. Oppenheimer JH, Koerner D, Schwartz HL, Surks MI 1972 Specific nuclear triiodothyronine binding sites in rat liver and kidney. J Clin Endocrinol Metab 35:330–333
4. Oppenheimer JH, Koerner D, Surks MI, Schwartz HL 1974 Limited binding capacity sites for L-triiodothyronine in rat liver nuclei: nuclear-cytoplasmic interrelationship, binding constants, and cross reactivity with L-thyroxine. J Clin Invest 53:768–777
5. DeGroot L, Strause J 1974 Binding of T3 in rat liver nuclei. Endocrinology 95:74–83
6. Samuels HH, Tsai JS 1973 Thyroid hormone action in cell culture: demonstration of nuclear receptors in intact cells and isolated nuclei. Proc Natl Acad Sci USA 70:3488–3492
7. Tata JR, Widnell CC 1966 Ribonucleic acid synthesis during the early action of thyroid hormones. Biochem J 98:604–620
8. Wolff E, Wolff J 1964 The mechanism of action of thyroid hormones in the thyroid grand. In: Pitt-Rivers R, Trotter W. Butterworths, London, pp 237–282
9. Tata J 1974 Growth and developmental action of thyroid hormones at the cellular level. In: Greer M, Solomon D (ed) American Physiological Society, Washington, DC, pp 469–476

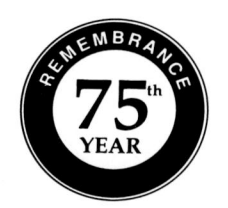

Remembrance: Discovery of the Vitamin D Endocrine System

Although the steroid nature of vitamin D should have suggested its hormonal nature, its discovery as a vitamin led to an expectation that it might act like other vitamins, *i.e.* as enzymatic cofactors. The first crack in this concept came when it became clear that the vitamin D molecule must be modified before it could function to elevate blood calcium, a discovery resulting from early metabolic work using chemically synthesized radiolabeled vitamin D_3 of high specific activity (1). This led to the discovery of the liver produced 25-hydroxyvitamin D_3 which for a time was believed to be the functional form of vitamin D_3 (2). Three laboratories contributed to the idea that 25-hydroxyvitamin D_3 is further metabolized before function (3–5). This metabolism occurs exclusively in the kidney (6). In 1970–1971, the active form of vitamin D was isolated from a target organ, the intestine, and chemically identified as $1\alpha,25$-dihydroxyvitamin D_3 (7). Chemical syntheses proved the 1-hydroxyl to be in the α-configuration (8). Thus, the active form of vitamin D originates in the kidney but has its function in intestine and bone. Therefore, $1\alpha,25$-dihydroxyvitamin D_3 must be considered a hormone and the kidney as the endocrine gland. Most important was the discovery that the production of $1\alpha,25$-dihydroxyvitamin D_3 is feedback regulated by serum calcium (9) through the parathyroid glands (10–12), clearly defining the vitamin D-based endocrine system. The full impact of this endocrine system is currently widely explored as is the molecular mechanism of action of $1\alpha,25$-dihydroxyvitamin D_3 and its regulation. Certainly the finding of a role for $1\alpha,25$-dihydroxyvitamin D_3 in differentiation, the immune system, reproduction, and other systems demonstrate the far-reaching importance of this recently arrived endocrine system.

Hector F. DeLuca
Department of Biochemistry
University of Wisconsin—Madison

Received October 3, 1991.
"Remembrance" articles discuss people and events as remembered by the author. The opinion(s) expressed are solely those of the writer and do not reflect the view of the Journal or The Endocrine Society.

References

1. Lund J, DeLuca HF 1966 Biologically active metabolite of vitamin D_3 from bone, liver, and blood serum. J Lipid Res 7:739–744
2. Blunt JW, DeLuca HF, Schnoes HK 1968 25-Hydroxycholecalciferol: a biologically active metabolite of vitamin D_3. Biochemistry 7:3317-3322
3. DeLuca HF 1970 Metabolism and function of vitamin D. In: DeLuca HF, Suttie JW (eds), The Fat-Soluble Vitamins. University of Wisconsin Press, Madison, pp 3–20
4. Lawson DEM, Wilson PW, Kodicek E 1969 Metabolism of vitamin D. A new cholecalciferol metabolite, involving loss of hydrogen at C-1, in chick intestinal nuclei. Biochem J 115:269–277
5. Haussler MR, Myrtle JF, Norman AW 1968 The association of a metabolite of vitamin D_3 with intestinal mucosa chromatin *in vivo*. J Biol Chem 243:4055–4064
6. Fraser DR, Kodicek E 1970 Unique biosynthesis by kidney of a biologically active vitamin D metabolite. Nature 228:764–766
7. Holick MF, Schnoes HK, DeLuca HF, Suda T, Cousins RJ 1971 Isolation and identification of 1,25-dihydroxycholecalciferol. A metabolite of vitamin D active in intestine. Biochemistry 10:2799–2804
8. Semmler EJ, Holick MF, Schnoes HK, DeLuca HF 1972 The synthesis of $1\alpha,25$-dihydroxycholecalciferol: a metabolically active form of vitamin D_3. Tetrahedron Lett 40:4147–4150
9. Boyle IT, Gray RW, DeLuca HF 1971 Regulation by calcium of *in vivo* synthesis of 1,25-dihydroxycholecalciferol and 21,25-dihydroxycholecalciferol. Proc Natl Acad Sci USA 68:2131–2134
10. Garabedian M, Holick MF, DeLuca HF, Boyle IT 1972 Control of 25-hydroxycholecalciferol metabolism by the parathyroid glands. Proc Natl Acad Sci USA 69:1673–1676
11. Fraser DR, Kodieck E 1973 Regulation of 25-hydroxycholecalciferol-1-hydroxylase activity in kidney by parathyroid hormone. Nature 241:163–166
12. Garabedian M, Tanaka Y, Holick MF, DeLuca HF 1974 Response of intestinal calcium transport and bone calcium mobilization to 1,25-dihydroxyvitamin D_3 in thyroparathyroidectomized rats. Endocrinology 94:1022–1027

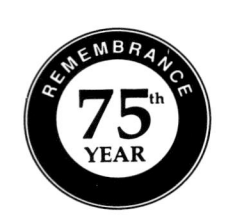

Remembrance: Steps Leading to the Identification, Purification, and Characterization of the Glucocorticoid Receptor

My work on glucocorticoid action and receptor structure and function started indirectly upon my return from a postdoctoral fellowship at the Biochemical Laboratories of the Sorbonne in Paris in 1954, where I worked on lysozyme and also on the mechanism of protease action. After being informed by the Office of Naval Research that I would not have to serve out my military obligation, I accepted the position of assistant professor at Rutgers University and had decided, while I was still in Paris, that I wanted to work on hormone action. I chose as a model the GH stimulation of the rat levator ani muscle. Soon after I switched my attention from the levator ani muscle to liver enzymes with the same control system in mind. In those days, preparations of GH obtainable through an NIH program were still contaminated with TSH. Animals treated with T_4 as a control for the TSH contamination in GH were studied. In 1956, I found some interesting effects of thyroid hormone on the tyrosine oxidation system, specifically with the initial enzyme of the pathway, tyrosine aminotransferase. I continued this work on thyroid hormone effects in this system and after moving to the University of Pennsylvania in 1960, I was impressed by the work of Knox and Mehler who showed that tyrosine aminotransferase was one of two liver enzymes induced by glucocorticoids. I became interested in what might be the mechanism of this induction. Thanks to the availability of [^{14}C]cortisol, I was able to study the intracellular fate of this isotopically labeled substance and provided evidence for cytoplasmic to nuclear translocation in 1963, although I did not appreciate the significance of those data at that time.

In that same year I attempted to study the earliest effects of the hormone by injecting [^{14}C]cortisol into rats and determining the fates of this labeled material in liver. The earliest time I could make observations was about 2 min after injection of the isotope. What I found under these conditions was macromolecular binding of the radioactivity and I proceeded to separate and study the macromolecules in work carried out at the Fels Institute for Cancer Research and Molecular Biology starting in 1964. Some proteins turned out to be bound with metabolites of cortisol and others bound the unmetabolized hormone. The most abundant protein was studied first. It bound both unmetabolized cortisol and its disulfate derivative. This protein was found to be identical to the principal azo dye binding protein of liver and the liver bilirubin binding protein and was named "ligandin" by the laboratories of Ketterer, Arias, and myself. Later, it was demonstrated to be the glutathione S-transferase system, a major protective mechanism against xenobiotics in the liver. Members of this highly concentrated (*c.a.* 4% of liver cytosol) family contain a binding pocket responsible for binding a wide variety of compounds, hence the original name, ligandin.

Next, my laboratory tackled the unmetabolized cortisol binding protein that we reported in 1973 to be the glucocorticoid receptor. We were able to define it as the receptor protein from the other four proteins involved as either metabolite binding proteins or parental hormone binding proteins. Primarily, this characterization rested on the ability to bind native hormone, reflect appropriate preference for steroidal ligands, saturate hormone binding at levels expected for the glucocorticoid levels, translocate to the nucleus, concentrate at low levels in the cell approaching that expected of the steroid, and complete its action well before the induction of liver enzymes. The other proteins were before or subsequently shown by us to be ligandin, a protein of about 10,000 Daltons reminiscent of growth factors, Binder 1B which we now believe occurs through an internal start site of the glucocorticoid receptor gene, and the 14,000 Daltons fatty acid binding protein known then as the "z protein." We purified the receptor protein as best we could in those days by gel filtration, ion exchange chromatography, and by preparative isoelectric focusing. We identified two major forms of the receptor as the unactivated and activated forms and we published the separation of these forms on diethylaminoethyl Sephadex.

Considerably before this, interestingly enough, we had performed what was probably the first "hot plus cold"

Received August 13, 1991.
"Remembrance" articles discuss people and events as remembered by the author. The opinion(s) expressed are solely those of the writer and do not reflect the view of the Journal or The Endocrine Society.

isotopically labeled glucocorticoid experiment, except that it was carried out *in vivo*, which gave an idea of specific binding. This earlier work may have contributed to the commonly used hot plus cold experiment *in vitro* for the determination of specific receptor binding activity.

We were also able to extract the nuclear form of the receptor and characterize it by both ion exchange and gel filtration chromatography. There appeared to be two separable forms of the nuclear receptor. By 1973, we were able to clearly define and present a partial purification of the glucocorticoid receptor from liver. Subsequently in 1984, we reported, I think, the first purification to near homogeneity of the unactivated (non-DNA binding) form of the oligomeric receptor complex and showed that two proteins might accompany the receptor in this complex. We failed to provide early evidence for the presence of HSP90 since, in our hands, HSP90 was dissociated from the complex in the initial affinity purification step (this mysteriously occurred without a noticeable change in the apparent molecular weight compared to that of the cytosolic complex). However, our laboratory was the first to show a metal content of the receptor and based on experiments with phenanthroline, we postulated the metal to be zinc. Having the means to purify the non-DNA-binding receptor complex enabled the elaboration of the *in vitro* activation mechanism which we reported in 1985. This could now be coupled with earlier work on receptor regulators, such as modulator. Two modulators subsequently have been found and appear to be novel glycerophosphate derivatives. At least one of these may bridge the receptor to nonhomologous proteins in the unactivated complex. Recently, these modulators have been shown to be superactivators of protein kinase C, a finding that may provide the basis for coupling cell membrane events with the cytoplasmic receptor system. Finally, the receptor has been overexpressed in insect cells so as to provide large amounts for further characterization and determination of three-dimensional structure.

The beginnings of this work occurred at a time, around 1960–1965 when there had been little thought of the existence of receptors. Unfortunately, we were unaware of the early work of Jensen and his collaborators that was going on at about the same time when his laboratory was involved in studying the specific uptake and retention of estradiol by various tissues. This period marked a turning point in the thinking about hormone action which up to then was considered to involve direct effects of hormones upon enzymes. Forthcoming work will complete the receptor mechanism and three-dimensional structure, a remarkable progression in three short decades.

Gerald Litwack
Department of Pharmacology and the
  Jefferson Cancer Institute
Thomas Jefferson University

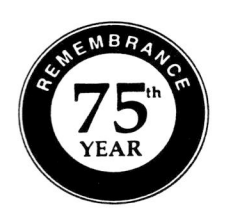

Remembrance: Scientific Contributions of Larry L. Ewing (1936–1990)

Dr. Larry Ewing died unexpectedly on August 13, 1990 near his home in Monkton, Maryland. At the time of his death at age 54, Larry was Professor, Division of Reproductive Biology, The Johns Hopkins University School of Hygiene and Public Health. Measured against any standard, Larry was a creative, highly productive investigator in male reproductive biology; an outstanding mentor; a leader in the scientific community; and perhaps most importantly, a dear friend to many of us. This brief chapter will highlight some of his major scientific contributions, and will provide a glimpse into the personal qualities that he brought to his work.

Larry was born on a farm in Valley, Nebraska on July 10, 1936. After graduating with a B.S. from the School of Agriculture of the University of Nebraska in 1958, he began predoctoral study in reproductive physiology in the Department of Dairy Science, University of Illinois. Four years later, in 1962, he received the Ph.D. degree. One of the papers (1) that resulted from his thesis research, entitled "Factors Affecting Testicular Metabolism and Function. I. A Simplified Perfusion Technique for Short-Term Maintenance of Rabbit Testis," set a major tone for his life-long interest in the regulation of the biosynthetic properties and structure of the Leydig cell in the mammalian testis.

Immediately upon the completion of the Ph.D. program, Larry, then age 26, joined the faculty of Oklahoma State University as an Assistant Professor in the Department of Physiology and Pharmacology. While at Oklahoma State, he began what was to be a long, fruitful collaboration with Dr. Claude Desjardins on the effects of steroid feedback on spermatogenesis. Ewing and Desjardins demonstrated for the first time that the administration of steroid (testosterone) to rabbits via sustained release Silastic capsules could cause azoospermia (2). Later, with Desjardins and Dr. Bernard Robaire, these initial observations in the rabbit were extended to other mammalian species (rat, monkey) in which the administration of testosterone alone had failed to produce azoospermia. They demonstrated that a combination of testosterone and estradiol acted synergistically to profoundly suppress LH secretion, and thus produced consistent, reversible azoospermia (3, 4).

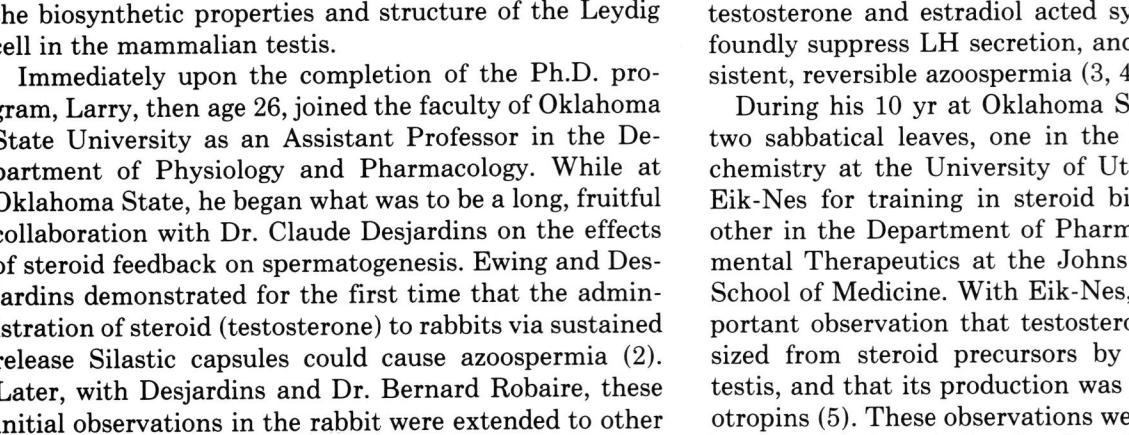

During his 10 yr at Oklahoma State, Larry arranged two sabbatical leaves, one in the Department of Biochemistry at the University of Utah with Dr. Kristen Eik-Nes for training in steroid biochemistry, and the other in the Department of Pharmacology and Experimental Therapeutics at the Johns Hopkins University School of Medicine. With Eik-Nes, Larry made the important observation that testosterone could be synthesized from steroid precursors by the perfused rabbit testis, and that its production was responsive to gonadotropins (5). These observations were central to many of his later studies relating Leydig cell structure and function.

In 1972, Larry, then age 35, was recruited to the Department of Population Dynamics as Professor and first Head of a newly constituted Division of Reproductive Biology. His productivity at Hopkins was truly remarkable. Among his many discoveries were the follow-

---

Received September 30, 1991.
"Remembrance" articles discuss people and events as remembered by the author. The opinion(s) expressed are solely those of the writer and do not reflect the view of the Journal or The Endocrine Society.

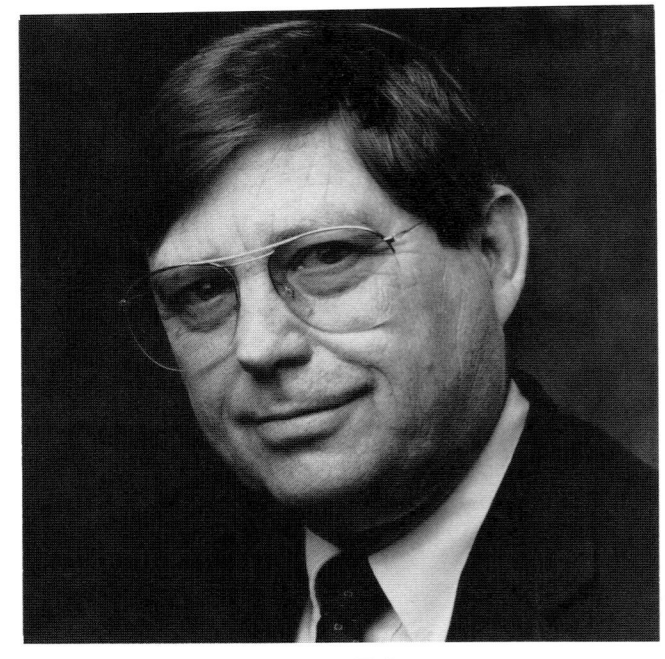

ing: 1) With Drs. Terry Turner and Stuart Howards, it was established that there is a downward gradient in testosterone concentration from the interstitial to the seminiferous tubular compartment of the testis, and that there is a rise in dihydrotestosterone concentration from the testis to the epididymis (6, 7). 2) With Drs. Stephen Berry (then a predoctoral student), Donald Coffey, and Patrick Walsh, convincing evidence was obtained that the dihydrotestosterone content of the dog and human hyperplastic prostatic tissue does not differ from that of control tissue (8–10). 3) With Drs. Curtis Chubb (then a predoctoral student) and Bernard Robaire, evidence was obtained that the diffusion of steroids from the Leydig cell is enhanced by steroid-binding macromolecules in the blood (11). 4) With Dr. Chubb, evidence was obtained for the existence of preferred testosterone biosynthetic pathways in different species (12). 5) With Dr. Barry Zirkin, it was discovered that there is a linear, positive correlation between the ability of Leydig cells to produce testosterone in response to LH and the quantity of Leydig cell smooth endoplasmic reticulum (13). Later, with Dr. Chamindrani Mendis-Handagama, a highly significant, positive linear correlation was also found between testosterone production and peroxisome surface area in the Leydig cell (14). 6) With Dr. Tung-Yang Wing, evidence was obtained that the quantity of Leydig cell smooth endoplasmic reticulum and the capacity of the testes to produce testosterone both depend upon LH; the conversion of pregnenolone to progesterone was found to be unaffected by LH, but the reactions responsible for converting progesterone to testosterone were found to be highly dependent upon LH (15). 7) With Drs. Diane Keeney (then a predoctoral student) and Mendis-Handagama, it was shown that although LH is required to maintain Leydig cell structure and function, it is not required to maintain Leydig cell number (16). 8) With Dr. Matthew Hardy, convincing evidence that Leydig cells differentiate from mesenchymal precursor cells during puberty was obtained (17). 9) With Dr. Gary Klinefelter, a new procedure was developed for the isolation of highly purified Leydig cells that were well preserved structurally and functionally (18). 10) With Drs. Klinefelter and Hardy and Dr. William Kelce, it was shown that the culture of isolated mesenchymal cells from prepubertal rats with a combination LH and dihydrotestosterone results in significant increases in the ability of the precursor cells to secrete testosterone, suggesting that androgens may regulate the differentiation of precursor cells to Leydig cells (19).

Simply put, Larry's contributions to our knowledge of Leydig cell structure, function, and regulation were remarkable. Moreover, he also distinguished himself as a teacher and administrator. A first-rate educator, he trained 32 students and fellows, and influenced countless others. He was one of the founders, and later the President, of the Society for the Study of Reproduction, and served as Editor-in-Chief of *Biology of Reproduction*. In 1987, he received the Distinguished Service Award of the Society for the Study of Reproduction. He also was President of the American Society of Andrology. He served on major committees of the Environmental Protection Agency, Food and Drug Administration, and National Academy of Sciences. He organized national meetings for the Society of the Study of Reproduction, American Society of Andrology, and the Testis Workshop.

Larry's achievements in research, teaching, and administration all stemmed from his unwillingness to accept less than excellence, and in his remarkable ability to interact with people and to make them feel special. He provided undivided attention to those with whom he interacted, always willing to share his expertise, his advice, his comfort, and his joy. His genuine interest in the persons with whom he interacted, and his enthusiasm for whatever he was listening to or arguing with, boosted the confidence and excitement of the young and the established alike. These qualities, together with his enormous integrity, stand as hallmarks of Larry Ewing's character and accomplishment. Neither he, nor his outstanding work, will soon be forgotten.

B. R. Zirkin
Division of Reproductive Biology
Department of Population Dynamics
The Johns Hopkins University
School of Hygiene and Public Health

References

1. VanDemark NL, Ewing LL 1963 Factors affecting testicular metabolism and function. I. A simplified perfusion technique for short-term maintenance of rabbit testis. J Reprod Fertil 6:1–6
2. Ewing LL, Stratton LG, Desjardins C 1973 Effect of testosterone polydimethylsiloxane implants upon sperm production, libido and accessory sex organ function in rabbits. J Reprod Fertil 35:245–253
3. Ewing LL, Desjardins C, Irby DC, Robaire B 1977 Synergistic interaction of testosterone and oestradiol inhibits spermatogenesis in rats. Nature 269:409–411
4. Robaire B, Ewing LL, Irby DC, Desjardins C 1979 Interactions of testosterone and estradiol-17β on the reproductive tract of the male rat. Biol Reprod 21:445–463
5. Ewing LL, Eik-Nes KB 1966 On the formation of testosterone by the perfused rabbit testis. Can J Biochem 44:1327–1344
6. Turner TT, Jones CE, Howards SS, Ewing LL, Zegeye B, Gunsalus GL 1984 On the androgen microenvironment of maturing spermatozoa. Endocrinology 115:1925–1932
7. Turner TT, Ewing LL, Jones CE, Howards SS, Zegeye B 1985 Androgens in male rat reproductive fluids: hypophysectomy and steroid replacement. Am J Physiol 248:E274–E280
8. Ewing LL, Berry SJ, Higginbottom EG 1983 Dihydrotestosterone concentration of beagle prostatic tissue: effect of age and hyperplasia. Endocrinology 113:2004–2009
9. Berry SJ, Coffey DS, Strandberg JD, Ewing LL 1986 Effect of age, castration and testosterone replacement on the development and restoration of canine benign prostatic hyperplasia. Prostate 9:295–302
10. Walsh PC, Hutchins GM, Ewing LL 1983 Tissue content of dihy-

drotestosterone in human prostatic hyperplasia is not supranormal. J Clin Invest 72:1772-1777
11. Ewing LL, Chubb CE, Robaire B 1976 Macromolecules, steroid binding and testosterone secretion by rabbit testes. Nature 264:84-86
12. Chubb C, Ewing LL 1979 Steroid secretion by *in vitro* perfused testes: testosterone biosynthetic pathways. Am J Physiol 237:E247-E254
13. Ewing LL, Zirkin B 1983 Leydig cell structure and steroidogenic function. Recent Prog Horm Res 39:599-635
14. Mendis-Handagama SMLC, Zirkin BR, Ewing LL 1988 Comparison of components of the testis interstitium with testosterone secretion in hamster, rat, and guinea pig testes perfused *in vitro*. Am J Anat 181:12-22
15. Wing T-Y, Ewing LL, Zirkin BR 1984 Effect of luteinizing hormone withdrawal on Leydig cell smooth endoplasmic reticulum and steroidogenic reactions which convert pregnenolone to testosterone. Endocrinology 115:2290-2296
16. Keeney DS, Mendis-Handagama SMLC, Zirkin BR, Ewing LL 1988 Effect of long term deprivation of luteinizing hormone on Leydig cell volume, Leydig cell number, and steroidogenic capacity of the rat testis. Endocrinology 123:2906-2915
17. Hardy MP, Zirkin BR, Ewing LL 1989 Kinetic studies on the development of the adult population of Leydig cells in testes of the pubertal rat. Endocrinology 124:762-770
18. Klinefelter GR, Hall PF, Ewing LL 1987 Effect of luteinizing hormone deprivation *in situ* on steroidogenesis of rat Leydig cells purified by a multistep procedure. Biol Reprod 36:769-783
19. Hardy MP, Kelce WR, Klinefelter GR, Ewing LL 1990 Differentiation of Leydig cell precursors *in vitro*: a role for androgen. Endocrinology 127:488-490

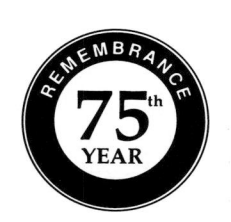

Remembrance: Neuroendocrinology and Aging. A Perspective

Brown-Sequard, the "father of endocrinology," was probably the first experimental gerontologist. He believed that testicular hormone secretion declined with age in men (as demonstrated many years later) and this led to a general decrease in body functions. In 1889 at the age of 72 yr, feeling that he was failing in physical and mental vigor, he injected himself with crushed dog and guinea pig testes to which a little water was added and passed through a Pasteur filter. He announced that this treatment reinvigorated him and that he could now work in his laboratory all day, and after dinner in the evening, could write and follow other mental pursuits. This aroused considerable skepticism among some but also led to many attempts to improve declining body functions by endocrine and other means which continue to the present day.

Early studies on hormone-aging relationships included measurements of changes in size and weight of endocrine glands and target organs, examination of alterations in their gross and microscopic appearance, bioassays of hormones in endocrine glands, blood, and urine, and clinical observations of endocrine related disorders in elderly individuals. The unavailability of RIAs for accurate measurement of hormone levels in the blood, and lack of knowledge of the commanding role of the hypothalamus in regulating pituitary and indirectly, target gland hormone secretion, greatly limited the scope of the early investigations, and little definitive information was forthcoming. This led several leading gerontological investigators (Korenchevsky, Verzar, and others) to conclude that hormones have only a minor role in aging processes. In light of present knowledge of the important involvement of the neuroendocrine system in aging processes, it can be stated that these conclusions were premature.

Studies on the relation of the neuroendocrine system to aging began in the 1960s and early 1970s. The first reports by Aschheim (1) in France, Peng (2) in Taiwan, and our laboratory (3) dealt with the relation of the hypothalamus to the reproductive decline in rats. Aschheim (1) showed that when ovaries from young rats were transplanted to old noncycling rats after ovariectomy, the old rats failed to exhibit estrous cycles. On the other hand, when ovaries from old noncycling female rats were transplanted to young ovariectomized rats, estrous cycles ensued in many of the young rats. Peng (2) confirmed these results, and also demonstrated that when the pituitary of old noncycling rats was removed and implanted underneath the median eminence of hypophysectomized young rats, many of the young rats resumed cycling. These important observations demonstrated that neither the ovaries nor the pituitary were mainly responsible for loss of cycling in aging rats, and suggested that cessation of cycling was probably due to faults that developed in the hypothalamus.

The first study to demonstrate direct hypothalamic involvement in loss of reproductive cycles in rats was our report in 1969 showing that electrical stimulation of the preoptic area induced ovulation in old constant estrous rats (3). Injections of epinephrine-in-oil or progesterone also resulted in ovulation. The observation that electrical stimulation of the preoptic area was effective suggested that sufficient LHRH was present in the hypothalamus to elicit LH release, but the stimulus for its release was lacking. The finding that epinephrine also was effective in evoking ovulation suggested that the missing stimulus might be a catecholamine (CA). Subsequently we found that both dopamine and norepinephrine were significantly reduced in the hypothalamus of old as compared to the amounts present in the hypothalamus of young rats (4–6). Administration of drugs that raised hypothalamic CAs, such as L-dopa, the precursor of CAs, or iproniazid, a monoamine oxidase inhibitor that depressed CA catabolism, induced resumption of estrous cycles in the old rats.

The decrease in hypothalamic dopamine activity in old rats and mice was found to be mainly responsible for the rise in PRL secretion and development of numerous mammary and PRL-secreting pituitary tumors. Administration of L-dopa or the longer acting ergot drugs that inhibit PRL secretion resulted in inhibition of PRL secretion and regression of mammary and pituitary tumors (5, 6). The reduction in hypothalamic CAs was also found to be responsible for the decline in GH and somatomedin-C secretion in old male and female rats (5–7). Injections of L-dopa were shown to return pulsatile GH secretion in old male rats to the same levels as in young male rats. In elderly man, a similar decline in GH

Received November 11, 1991.

"Remembrance" articles discuss people and events as remembered by the author. The opinion(s) expressed are solely those of the writer and do not reflect the view of the Journal or The Endocrine Society.

and somatomedin-C secretion was observed (8), and this too may be related to the reduction found in hypothalamic CAs (9). Administration of drugs that elevated hypothalamic CAs were reported by four different laboratories to significantly lengthen the average lifespan in rats or mice, decrease the incidence of disease and tumors, promote sexual vigor and fertility, and improve memory (see Ref. 6). These effects were not usually associated with reduced food intake or loss of body weight.

Other changes reported in the hypothalamus with age include loss of neurons in specific nuclei, a decrease in hormone receptors, an increase in hydrogen peroxide and hydroxyl radicals resulting from catabolism of CAs, a reduction in tyrosine hydroxylase, the rate-limiting enzyme for synthesis of CAs, and an increase in monoamine oxidase, the major enzyme responsible for catabolism of monoamines (see Refs. 5 and 6). These changes may largely account for the decline in hypothalamic CAs with age.

In addition to the dysfunctions that develop in the hypothalamus with age, there is evidence that other components of the neuroendocrine system develop faults. The pituitary of old rats has been reported to be less responsive to stimulation by GnRH, GHRH, TRH, and CRF than the pituitary of young rats (5, 6). Similarly the pituitary of elderly human subjects was observed to be less responsive to stimulation by GnRH and GHRH than the pituitary of young individuals (7, 10). There also is some evidence that target gland responses to pituitary hormones, and body tissue responses to target gland hormones may decrease with age. Some of these have been found to be associated with a decrease in receptors or to postreceptor changes in cells. These decreases in response of endocrine and nonendocrine tissues to hormones are believed to be of secondary importance to the faults that develop in the hypothalamus with age.

Significant declines also occur in the immune system with age. Since the neuroendocrine and immune systems function coordinately as a bidirectional network, and both systems exhibit a functional decline with age, it is important to determine the relation of each system to the decline of the other. There is evidence that the reduction in immune function with age is at least partly attributable to the decrease in GH and thyroid hormone secretion (11). Administration of GH to old rats was reported to return size and function of the thymus gland, the chief component of the immune system, to the same levels as in young rats (12). Administration of T_4 similarly elevated thymic function in old mice (11). The effects of the immune system on neuroendocrine function with age are presently unknown, but there is substantial evidence that thymic peptides can alter hypothalamic, pituitary, and target gland hormone secretion.

Most gerontological investigators agree that the genome is of primary importance in regulating length of life, which is related to aging, and that environmental factors are also involved. We believe that the genome and environment exert their effects on aging processes mainly via the neuroendocrine and immune systems, the two systems of the body which are most important for integrating body functions and maintaining homeostasis. Other theories have emphasized changes in transfer of information from DNA via mRNA resulting in errors in protein synthesis, an increase in "free radicals" with resulting damage to many body cells, a failure of cells to divide or function due to loss of a genetic program, *etc*. It is doubtful that any single theory of the causes of aging can explain all aspects of the aging phenomenon. It is clear however, that the neuroendocrine approach, although relatively recent in origin, has already provided some valuable knowledge and insights into the causes of the aging declines in body functions, and suggested methods of intervention that may inhibit or reverse aging processes and perhaps lengthen the lifespan.

Joseph Meites
Department of Physiology
Michigan State University

References

1. Aschheim P 1976 Aging in the hypothalamic hypophyseal ovarian axis in the rat. In: Everitt AV, Burgess JA (eds) Hypothalamus, Pituitary and Aging. Chas C Thomas, Springfield IL, p 376–418
2. Peng MT 1983 Changes in hormone uptake and receptors in the hypothalamus during aging. In: Meites J (ed) Neuroendocrinology of Aging. Plenum Press, New York, p 61–72
3. Clemens JA, Amenomori Y, Jenkins T, Meites J 1969 Effects of hypothalamic stimulation, hormones and drugs on ovarian function in old female rats. Proc Soc Exp Biol Med 132:561–563
4. Simpkins JW, Mueller JP, Huang HH, Meites J 1977 Evidence for depressed catecholamines and enhanced serotonin metabolism in aging male rats: possible reltion to gonadotropin secretion. Endocrinology 100:1672–1678
5. Meites J, Goya R, Takahashi S 1987 Why the neuroendocrine system is important in aging processes. Exp Gerontol 22:1–15
6. Meites J 1990 Aging: hypothalamic catecholamines, neurocrine-immune interactions, and dietary restriction. Proc Soc Exp Biol Med 195:304–311
7. Sonntag WE, Meites J 1988 Decline in growth hormone secretion in aging animals and man. In: Everitt AV, Walton JR (eds) Regulation of Neuroendocrine Aging. Karger AG, Basel, p 111–124
8. Florini JR, Prinz PN, Vitiello MV, Hintz RL 1985 Somatomedin-C levels in healthy young and old men: relationship to peak and 24-hour integrated levels of growth hormone. J Gerontol 40:2–7
9. Horniekiewicz O 1987 Neurotransmitter changes in human brain during aging. In: Govoni S, Battaini F (eds) Modifications of Cell to Cell Signals during Normal and Pathological Aging. Springer Verlag, Berlin, p 169–182
10. Harman SM 1978 Clinical aspects of aging of the male reproductive system. In: Schneider EL (ed) The Aging Reproductive System. Raven Press, New York, p 29–58
11. Fabris N, Mocchegiani E, Muzzioli M, Provenciali M 1988 Immuneneuroendocrine interactions during aging. Prog Neuroendocrinimmunol 1:4–9
12. Kelley KW, Brief S, Westley HJ, Novakofski J, Bechtel PJ, Simon J, Walker EB 1986 GH_3 pituitary adenoma cells can reverse thymic aging in rats. Proc Natl Acad Sci USA 83:5666–5667

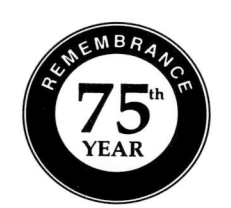

Remembrance: Tracing the Glucose Tracer Dilution Technique for Measuring Glucose Turnover

The technique using radioactive glucose to measure glucose production and uptake, first developed in animals and in the early 1970s applied to humans, is now used almost routinely in metabolic research units throughout the world. There were two milestones in the development of this technique which led to its wide acceptance. One was the introduction of the priming injection-constant infusion of the ^{14}C labeled glucose which simplified the technique and the second was the replacement of the ^{14}C label by ^{3}H, specifically at carbon 3 of the glucose, which opened its use in humans. Some of the events leading to these developments are offered as reflections in this presentation.

^{14}C-Labeled glucose was first used to measure the size of the glucose pool and rates of glucose turnover in rats, dogs, and humans in the early 1950s. It was commonly injected as a single iv bolus and from the changing ratio of the glucose $^{14}C/^{12}C(SA)$ in subsequent serial blood samples one could calculate the size of the glucose pool and turnover rate. There were shortcomings to this technique because a number of factors could influence the calculations. Thus, reincorporation of the ^{14}C released from the metabolized tracer into newly released glucose (recycling) would tip upward the slope of the falling specific activity and result in overestimation of the size of the glucose pool and underestimation of the turnover rate. Although such recycling of tracer could be corrected for by using glucose labeled in only one carbon, the single injection also gave wrong interpretations regarding endogenous glucose production when plasma glucose levels were changing rapidly in the course of the study. This is strikingly demonstrated in studies on the effect of a glucose load on glucose production. After the bolus injection of the tracer glucose and the consequent progressive fall in the plasma glucose specific activity, injection of an unlabeled glucose load would result in a prompt plateau in the glucose specific activity, which would last throughout the period of hyperglycemia and then commence to decline again upon restoration of normal plasma glucose levels. The plateau was interpreted to indicate a complete cessation of hepatic glucose release into the plasma. However, during a summer interlude with Rachmiel Levine at Brookhaven National Lab, Bob Steele and Jonathan Bishop (1) showed that, using a single injection of tracer glucose, a similar plateau in glucose specific activity could be demonstrated after a cold glucose load in eviscerated dogs, thus making untenable the interpretation that glucose production had been shut down by the glucose load.

As an alternative to the single injection of isotopic glucose, one could deliver the glucose by a constant infusion until the plasma glucose specific activity reached a plateau, which would simplify the calculation of glucose turnover. The limitation of this approach would be the 5–6 h required to reach the plateau and one still had the problem of calculating the size of the glucose pool. The limitations of each approach were appreciated by Gilbert Searle et al. (2), who used two experiments to calculate the pool and turnover rate. In the first experiment they injected a single dose of tracer glucose and used the fall of the glucose specific activity as a measurement of the ratio of glucose pool to turnover rate. Some 3 weeks later, using the same dog, they would administer the glucose tracer as a single bolus along with a constant infusion in a ratio calculated from the first experiment. The experiment was successful if they maintained a constant level of plasma specific activity beginning with the start of the second hour. Although such studies provided reliable data, it was obvious that a simpler approach would be desirable. Essentially, Robert Steele et al. (3) developed the calculations which allowed us to determine the glucose pool size and turnover rate in one experiment, rather than two, by infusing tracer glucose as a single or "priming" injection along with a constant infusion. This approach usually established a steady plasma glucose specific activity within 1 h, which allowed for blood sampling in the second hour to obtain control values, and thence to proceed with the various experimental protocols. A subsequent set of calculations was developed to determine rates of glucose production and uptake by tissues when rapid changes in plasma glucose were induced experimentally. This was necessary because of the slow mixing of the tracer glucose with the unlabeled glucose, be it endogenous or administered glucose. Using an electronic analog of a dog and some brief *in vivo* mixing

Received December 31, 1991.
"Remembrance" articles discuss people and events as remembered by the author. The opinion(s) expressed are solely those of the writer and do not reflect the view of the Journal or The Endocrine Society.

experiments, we concluded that there was a rapidly mixing compartment of glucose, which comprised approximately 50% of the total body glucose pool, including the plasma glucose (4). This number for the rapidly mixing pool was subsequently increased to 65% by the elegant studies of Cowan and Hetenyi (5). Use of either number, with appropriate control experiments, give essentially the same conclusions.

Apart from the calculations and interpretation of the data, the logistics of doing the experiment had presented a considerable challenge. Since the experiments were to be done without anesthesia, the dogs required several weeks of conditioning to lie quietly on an operating table. In addition, to allow collection of exhaled CO_2 and the ^{14}C it contained, we had to design comfortable and yet practical enclosures for the dog's head. We settled on a rigid plastic cylinder, about 10 in. in diameter. One end plate of the cylinder was removable and was in two parts, with a half circle cut out from each half so that the two parts could be enclosed around the dog's neck. To assure complete collection of the CO_2, a rubber sheet (dentist dam) was cemented around the dog's neck and that in turn was secured to the end plate. Air was drawn through the mask at 30 liters/min, and then through a flow meter and a vat containing 20 liters sodium hydroxide, which trapped all the CO_2 and the remainder was blown off into a hood. It was gratifying to see how well the dogs accepted the procedure and since the same dogs were used for a number of years, a strong bond was established between the subjects and the experimenters.

The first studies were carried out by Joseph Wall, Robert Steele, Richard deBodo, and myself at the New York University School of Medicine. Joe Wall was a chemist by training and actually spent several months at Brookhaven National Lab on Long Island to prepare the high specific activity, uniformly labeled [^{14}C]glucose. He exposed Canna leaves to an atmosphere of $^{14}CO_2$ and eventually isolated and extracted the radioactive glucose. We used this batch until good quality commercial sources became available. The blood sampling was also a laborious and anxiety producing step. This task was taken over by the senior member of our group, Richard deBodo, at his own insistence. To assure the timely sampling, the femoral artery was exposed, which involved initial cutdown and closing of the wound at the end of each experiment. Happily for deBodo and the dogs this ritual did not persist for too long, because with the arrival of David Armstrong as a post doc, we learned to insert a polyethylene tube into the vein percutaneously through a needle. We then routinely used this procedure for sampling from the jugular vein and infusion into the saphenous vein.

Analysis of the radioactivity in the plasma and CO_2 samples was another formidable task. The glucose was isolated as a phenylosazone derivative, which was subsequently combusted to CO_2 using the Van Slyke and Folch wet combustion method. The CO_2 was then transferred to the gas phase proportional counter for measuring the ^{14}C in a β-counter. The proportional counters were cylindrical tubes, nearly a meter long with a 2-cm diameter and the inner walls covered with silver. The complete transfer of the ^{14}C from the combustion chamber to the counter involved opening and closing a number of stop cocks and lowering and raising a heavy reservoir of mercury. Since this procedure was carried out on each sample, our female technicians made the workup into a exercise ritual and developed a most enviable set of bicep and tricep muscles. The entire preparation of each sample for counting required at least 15 min but all this was soon supplanted by the development of a glucosotriazole derivative of the isolated glucose which could be counted easily by liquid scintillation.

We presented our first data at the 1955 Federation meeting, at the magnificent Malborough Blenheim hotel in Atlantic City. At the time there was considerable controversy as to why the hypophysectomized animal had lower than normal blood glucose levels. Jane Russell, who was a highly regarded and well established investigator, believed that the lower blood glucose levels in these animals were due to increased glucose use, based on the fact that such operated rats disposed of a cold glucose load more rapidly than did normal rats. Others who measured A-V differences across the liver held that the operated animals had lower glucose values because they produced less glucose. Our data showed that hypophysectomized dogs had lower rates of glucose production and use in the basal state. I was most excited to present such clear findings obtained for the first time with this new elegant technique and this was to be my first presentation at a Federation meeting. My enthusiasm abated rather abruptly when I looked out at the audience and saw Dr. Russell sitting smack in from of me. As expected, the data were challenged on the basis of newness of the technique. Our conclusions were amply confirmed, but the recollection of the encounter still evokes a strong sympathetic discharge.

While the priming injection-constant infusion of [^{14}C] glucose was used extensively in animals, it was not extended to humans presumably because of the concern about the potential dangers of ^{14}C accumulation in tissues. Consequently attention turned to the use of ^{3}H as the radiolabel for glucose. There were many advantages to the use of tritiated glucose. The plasma glucose did not have to be isolated directly since the ^{3}H in the plasma was contained mainly in glucose and water. Thus the plasma samples were deproteinized and an aliquot of each filtrate would be evaporated to eliminate the tritiated water, leaving only the radioactive glucose to be counted directly. Another advantage was that any ^{3}H released from the metabolized labeled glucose would be diluted by the huge mass of body water thus eliminating recycling of the label as a concern. And last, the ^{3}H would be eliminated readily from the body making it a more practical tracer for use in humans.

The first significant use of tritiated glucose for glucose turnover studies in whole animals was by Katz and Dunn (6). Arnold Dunn, who spent 6 yr with us before going to University of Southern California in 1962, decided to pursue his research interests in rats and with Joe Katz, who had extensive experience with ^{3}H, published their first paper on the use of tritiated glucose in 1967 (6). This study did not result in a prompt switch of isotopes by the various groups doing tracer metabolic studies in whole animals and it was not until 1972 that the first papers appeared using tritiated glucose in sheep (7) and dogs (8). About that time, we too had become interested in using tritiated glucose. Bob Steele had gone off on a year long sabbatical on the West coast and a recent graduate, Amiram Barkai, arrived in my lab and together we began to explore the use of tritiated glucose in our dogs. Katz and Dunn, in their initial study and later ones in 1974 (9), indicated that [2^{3}H]glucose was the appropriate isotope for such metabolic studies. They found that glucose turnover in the rat was about 1.5 times higher when using [2^{3}H]glucose than with [U^{14}C]glucose and they attributed the lower values to recycling of the ^{14}C label. Similar findings were reported in the dog by the Bela Issekutz group (8) and they too attributed the lower values for glucose turnover to recycling of the ^{14}C although they had no direct evidence for it.

In our initial experiments we were concerned about the issue of ^{14}C recycling and therefore compared glucose turnover values obtained with [2^{3}H] glucose *vs.* [6^{14}C] glucose. We selected this specific ^{14}C label so that we could correct for any recycling of ^{14}C. Our caution was well founded because the [2^{3}H]glucose tracer still gave us higher values for glucose turnover than with the [6^{14}C] glucose, so we were quite convinced that the discrepancy was not due to recycling of the ^{14}C, but perhaps was due to the choice of the tritiated label. We decided to use three different glucose tracers in the same experiment to compare the glucose turnover values. We compared [2^{3}H] glucose *vs.* [3^{3}H]glucose *vs.* [6^{14}C]glucose, the latter allowing correction for recycling of ^{14}C. Separation of tritium located at the C_2 position from that in the C_3 position in order to calculate their individual specific activities might seem like a forbidding task but it turned out to be very simple. We fell back on our standard technique for isolating glucose for scintillation counting of the radioactivity. The formation of glucosazone by the addition of phenylhydrazine to glucose removes ^{3}H only from the C_2 position, without affecting the ^{3}H at C_3.

Thus one could count total radioactivity in the glucose sample, then determine the radioactivity in the glucose derivative which is due to [3^{3}H]glucose and, by subtraction from the total radioactivity, obtain the radioactivity due to [2^{3}H]glucose. Determination of the radioactivity due to ^{14}C glucose followed routine steps and was independent of the tritium analysis.

The results of the foregoing experiments were very striking and unequivocal. They showed that [3^{3}H]glucose gave turnover values that were the same as those obtained with 6[^{14}C]glucose, corrected for recycling, whereas [2^{3}H]glucose gave turnover values that were about 40% higher (10). The higher values obtained with [2^{3}H]glucose are believed to reflect the different metabolic fates of the hydrogens on the various carbons of the glucose molecule. Hydrogen from the C_2 of glucose is lost in the reversible interconversion step between glucose-6-P and fructose-6-P. With [2^{3}H]glucose, the tritium at C^2 is lost to a greater extent than the tritium lost from C^3 when using [3^{3}H]glucose. A greater loss of tracer would be calculated as a greater turnover of glucose. Actually one may view the values obtained with [2^{3}H] glucose as approximating total glucose output and those obtained with [3^{3}H]glucose as measuring net glucose output. The difference in glucose turnover values using the two tracers has been used by several groups as a measure of glucose futile cycle activity.

We concluded from the above studies that [3^{3}H]glucose, rather than [2^{3}H]glucose, was the appropriate tracer to determine glucose turnover. Although this challenged the proposition that [2^{3}H]glucose was the appropriate tracer, submission of our data to Joe Katz persuaded him to accept our interpretation. I submitted the manuscript to the *Journal of Clinical Investigation* but it was not accepted for publication because it seemed to be just another glucose tracer for measuring glucose turnover and one was already available. Curiously, although Joe Katz was one of their reviewers and in the best position to evaluate our data, he was not asked to review the manuscript. I wrote a gentle and enlightening letter to the editor of *JCI* and submitted the paper early in November 1974 to the *American Journal of Physiology*. After waiting for several months, I had to call the Editor about the delay. When we finally received the comments of the one laggard reviewer, the strongest critique was that we did not use a least squares program to calculate the glucose specific activity asymptote, but rather depended on eyeballing it. It must have been evident to that reviewer that eyeballing a straight line was probably as reliable as any statistical program and that any discrepancy would be of little biologic significance. Nevertheless, with the aid of two colleagues, Bernard Altshuler and Naomi Harley, we developed a least squares computer solution, and I resubmitted the paper. Again there was a long wait and I was told that no decision would be made before the FASEB Federation meeting to be held in April 1975. Luckily we had submitted an abstract on these studies to that meeting, because we were chosen to present the material at a session devoted to isotopic studies of glucose and all the tracer officionados were there. Gene Yates was the session chairman and he was also the editor handling our manuscript. He told me just before the session that the fate of our paper would be determined by this meeting. Being a little more seasoned than during my earlier initiation rites and the encounter with Jane Russell, I rose to the occasion and gave an eloquent (so I was told) presentation of our work. The discussion that followed was most supportive. Arnold Dunn, who also presented a paper, graciously accepted our conclusion regarding the preference of [^{3}H]glucose for turnover studies. A challenging question from the audience suggesting the possibility that our tracer was being laid down in the outer chains of glycogen and rereleased as labeled glucose, thus leading to underestimation of glucose production, was disposed of promptly by Alan Cherrington, who had direct measurements of hepatic glucose output.

The meeting generated a great deal of excitement and in due time our paper was accepted for publication. It was submitted in early November 1974 and appeared in the December 1975 issue of the *American Journal of Physiology* (10). It is sobering to wonder how much would have had to be undone if this study had been denied publication. At any rate, this tracer technique was promptly applied to human studies and with innovative additions by numerous investigators, it continues to be a useful tool in metabolic studies.

Norman Altszuler
Department of Pharmacology
New York University School of Medicine

References

1. Steele R, Bishop JS, Levine R 1959 Does a glucose load inhibit hepatic sugar output? C^{14} glucose studies in eviscerated dogs. Am J Physiol 197(1):60–62
2. Searle GL, Strisower EH, Chaikoff IL 1954 Glucose pool and glucose space in the normal and diabetic dog. Am J Physiol 176:190–194
3. Steele R, Wall JS, deBodo RC, Altszuler N 1956 Measurement of size and turnover rate of body glucose pool by the isotope dilution method. Am J Physiol 187:15–24
4. Wall JS, Steele R, deBodo RC, Altszuler N 1957 Effect of insulin on utilization and production of circulating glucose. Am J Physiol 189:43–50
5. Cowan JS, Hetenyi Jr G 1971 Glucoregulatory responses in normal and diabetic dogs recorded by a new tracer method. Metabolism 20:360–372
6. Katz J, Dunn A 1967 Glucose-2-T as a tracer for glucose metabolism. Biochemistry 6:1–5
7. Judson GJ, Leng RA 1972 Estimation of the total entry rate and resynthesis of glucose in sheep using glucose uniformly labelled with ^{14}C and variously labelled with ^{3}H. Aust J Biol Sci 25:1313–1332
8. Issekutz Jr B, Allen M, Borkow I 1972 Estimation of glucose turnover in the dog with glucose-2-T and glucose-U-^{14}C. Am J Physiol 222:710–712
9. Katz J, Dunn A, Chenoweth M, Golden S 1974 Determination of synthesis, recycling and body mass of glucose in rats and rabbits *in vivo* with ^{3}H and ^{14}C-labelled glucose. Biochem J 142:171–183
10. Altszuler N, Barkai A, Bjerknes C, Gottlieb, Steele, R 1975 Glucose turnover values in the dog obtained with various species of labeled glucose. Am J Physiol 229(6):1662–1667

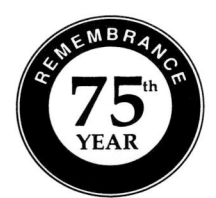

Remembrance: Mort and Griff

Mort Lipsett and Griff Ross were leaders in the study of reproductive endocrinology. Their work spanned a period of two decades and encompassed the years of the Vietnam war. They worked in the intramural program of the NIH. Mort was Chief, and Griff "Associate" Chief, of the Endocrinology Branch of the National Cancer Institute. The branch moved to the National Institute of Child Health and Human Development in 1970 and was renamed the Endocrinology and Reproduction Research Branch. Mort handled the paperwork. He was a superb administrator. The process was "clean" and efficient; everything up front, no hidden agendas, no deferred decisions, no looking back or second guessing. Griff handled the clinical responsibilities. He was a consummate physician; rounds every day, every problem considered, every patient talked to. He understood that "the cure commences when the eye of the patient meets the eye of the physician." Mort and Griff divided their scientific activities along "structural" lines. Mort worked with steroids; Griff with the gonadotropins. Interestingly, Mort, who disdained much of the medical process as "soft," did his greatest work on steroid metabolic interconversions in human subjects. Griff, who revered the practice of medicine, did his greatest work on the mechanisms of follicle growth and atresia in the rat. They worked together in harmony for more than 20 yr. Toward the end of his life, Mort told me that he and Griff never had an argument.

The two men had very different backgrounds. Mort was born in the Bronx of Jewish immigrant parents. His father was a pharmacist on 180th street. The family moved to San Francisco at the beginning of World War II. Mort went to "Berkeley" and majored in chemistry. His education was interrupted by the draft. He served as a Medic in the 10th Mountain Division and was twice decorated for valor in combat during the Italian campaign. After the war, he went to USC Medical school on the GI Bill. An internship at the L.A. County Hospital was followed by a medicine residency at the Sawtelle V.A. Hospital. Mort then returned to New York to work with Olaf Pearson at the Sloan Kettering. His interest in the endocrinology of neoplasia led to a position at the NIH with Roy Hertz. That was 1957. Mort was a genius. He forgot nothing, could beat three or four competent chess players at a time, was a life master bridge player, and could do differential equations in his head. He read articles vertically, and could toss off whole journals before the rest of us had finished the first few pages. When I tell this to people, they smile and consider it a gross exaggeration. All the more remarkable! Mort loved competition. He was focused on the state of his cardiovascular health. He relished a game of his own design, racing up 10 flights of stairs, and then seeing who could first decelerate their pulse to 60 beats/min or less. The younger the adversary, the better. Some of us never got down to a pulse of 60. Some of us never got to the 10th floor. Mort's taste in music ran to Mozart; in literature, to Thucidides and Gibbon; in art to Miro; in furniture, to Danish Modern; in food, to French; and in drink, to fine reds from the continent. Mort loved books. He used books like an artist uses brushes. He always had a book in hand. He left several of his endocrine texts to me. The gold lettering is worn off the covers by hard use, but the pages are clean; no marginalia, no dog ears. He treated books with respect, with a caress.

Griff was born in Mount Enterprise, East Texas. (He thought of East Texas as different from the larger entity. He called it the land of tall pines, red dirt, hook worm, and pellagra.) He came from Calvinist stock. He went to Stephen F. Austin State Teachers College and, in 1942, to the University of Texas Medical Branch in Galveston. He entered private practice in his hometown, the fourth generation of his family to do so. He was drafted into the Air Force with the Korean War and spent 2 yr as a general medical officer at an air base in England. When the war was over, Griff took a "Fellowship" in Internal Medicine at the "Mayo Brothers" clinic. Working with Al Albert, he developed a bioassay for urinary gonadotropins. This was the perfect tool for following the treatment response of patients with choriocarcinoma, and Griff came to the NIH 3 yr after Mort. Griff read slowly. He liked to "feel" his way through a problem. He disliked competition more intense than a friendly game of golf with wife and friends. He once told me that he belonged to "exercisers' anonymous." This was a mutual support group composed of a few close friends. If a member got the urge to exercise, he could call another member who would come and drink with him until the notion passed. Griff's taste in music ran to Bluegrass; in literature, to Steinbeck and Fitzgerald; in art, to Norman Rockwell; in furniture, to early American; in food, to Texas Bar-B-Que; and in drink, to martinis without Vermouth. Griff loved to make music. He played "by ear" and couldn't read music. None the less, he played saxophone in his college band, was an accomplished accordionist, and had a bagful of harmonicas, one in each key, that he played at every opportunity. He played hard; he is the only man I know who could "wear out" a harmonica. On the surface of things, the only way that Mort and Griff were alike was in their houses. But that was artifact since there was only one kind of house in Bethesda.

Mort and Griff were the beneficiaries of an accident of fate destined to change modern biomedical history; the contemporaneous opening of the Clinical Center at the NIH with the intensification on the Vietnam war. Physicians were

---

Received December 13, 1991.

"Remembrance" articles discuss people and events as remembered by the author. The opinion(s) expressed are solely those of the writer and do not reflect the view of the Journal or The Endocrine Society.

needed to manage research patients in the Clinical Center. The Public Health Service was the obvious source. Duty at the NIH became the only form of "alternate" military service at a time when most male graduates of American medical schools were being drafted. The NIH had its pick of the best that American medical education could offer. Thousands applied; 55 were chosen. These were the famous "Yellow Berets." They were distributed into subspecialties that many would never have considered under other circumstances. With a taste of success in research, they stayed. Rheumatology, infectious disease, endocrinology, and other cognitive specialties were peopled by young men of great promise. Women, not subject to the draft, rarely if ever came to the NIH by this mechanism. This, more than any other factor, accounts for the rarity of women from this generation in leadership positions in academic medicine.

Mort and Griff had different working styles. Mort would not spend time in conversation unless it was productively centered about a problem of interest. Even then, he wouldn't give it much effort unless there were new data. If there were, things happened fast. In his impatience to digest the material, he would take the data sheets from you. He worked best if you were quiet. This was learned quickly. You could follow Mort's progress through the data by the location of his index finger which moved with his eye. A quantitative analysis would begin as he approached the end. "This means. . . . ," or "remember that table in. . . ." A JCEM or JCI would be pulled from the shelf. Tables and isolated statements would be found with pinpoint accuracy. He would copy numbers out of these references, and make mental calculations. There was some conversation, but it was with himself, not you. Presently, comments and suggestions were made, and you were left to think it over alone in the library, books open everywhere, and a vague impression that instructions had been given. It could take hours to piece it together. The motivation was high, however, since nobody wanted to appear stupid. Twenty years later, I still occasionally "see", for the first time, what Mort was trying to tell me at some of those meetings. Mort was "deductively" hypertrophied. He moved fast with syllogisms, blindingly fast. He had no patience for doing it twice. He cut the path; you made the road.

Griff liked to "worry" the data. He would painstakingly study every number, asking question after question about the circumstances surrounding this particular experiment, or that outlier. He would recopy the numbers, rearrange them, "metabolize" them; there were no quick conclusions, no surgical insights. He would talk about the experiments for days. He would incorporate data from many sources and build a testable hypothesis. Griff was "Darwinian" in his reasoning; "inductively" hypertrophied. Mort left you shaken; Griff left you exhausted. Together, they "synergized."

Mort was free of preconception and bias; freer than any person I have known. He drove the scientific method into every recess of his life and ferreted out the last vestiges of dogma. He was free to see clearly. I well remember my first patient presentation to him. I had been warned to be ready with a thorough understanding of the nuances of the steroid abnormalities that were salient features of the case. I got through the tough part unscathed. In fact, Mort seemed bored by the whole thing. Wrapping up, I mentioned that because of an elevated postprandial glucose I had instructed the patient in a 1200 calorie diet and prescribed a distribution of calories recommended by the ADA. Mort woke up. "Why did you do that? Is there any evidence that this will help the man? Who does the cooking? His wife? How will this impact upon her? How much will it cost? What about the quality of life?" It went on. At the end, all I could muster was a weak "Well, this is the way that we did it at the Mecca." Mort, who by this time was half out of the door, retraced his steps. "This is the Mecca," he said. Mort wasn't angry (although it took years to understand that); he was merely illustrating an important point about the practice of medicine. He detested appeal to authority. In fact, no issue was too small to be unimportant in this way. Mort weighed facts in "Russelian" isolation where all were given equal weight. This clarity of process gave him great critical power. At the same time, it denied him a certain passion in science. Mort never loved a hypothesis.

Griff, on the other hand, held on to a hypothesis until it was dead by all accounts. Even then he would abandon it grudgingly. He would often return to the burial site looking for signs of life. Hypotheses came to Griff by a different process. Mort tended to engage problems of opportunity; Griff tended to "force the issue" with problems he considered to be of great importance. Hypotheses were hard won and precious. While Mort thought in mathematical abstractions, Griff thought in analogs. He made mental pictures of systems and thought about things in familiar terms (butter churns and hay balers were favorites). Like a young lover, Griff could overlook the most glaring defects in an idea because the rest of it was so beautiful. He would spend hours justifying the defect to whomever he could corner. When Griff had a new passion, word of it would pass quickly through the halls. People would begin to avoid him if they could; the slightest opening could lead to a prolonged discussion of the new idea. Out of respect and a certain sense of awe, nobody, once cornered, absented themselves until the event was over. A friend of mine shared an office with Griff and was easy prey because of proximity. Out of self-defense, he mastered the ability to divert his psychic energies to other problems during these dilations. He could "cut away" from the developing argument completely and yet maintain the appearance of engaged concentration. If Griff noticed, he never said so.

Griff was a "close range" doctor. He loved the history and physical examination. He loved best physical findings and their implications. I remember particularly the presentation of a short girl that Griff, in the course of the history, became convinced had Turner's syndrome. From that point onward, after the demonstration of each finding, Griff would say, "This is a sign of Turner's syndrome," and then explain why. At the end of the presentation it became clear that the girl did not have Turner's syndrome. Griff, unfazed, muttered, "we must never forget that all signs fail in dry weather!"

Mort and Griff tried life apart for a while. Mort had

expected, in time, to be appointed director of NICHD. When it failed to happen and the job was given to someone else, Mort decided that his future at the NIH was constricted. He left to head a Cancer Center in Cleveland. Griff became the Branch Chief in his stead and, in short order, was further burdened with the duties of Clinical and Scientific Director. The Cancer Center never really got off the ground and Mort was expected to be a Professor of Medicine in the traditional sense. His skepticism was misinterpreted as lack of knowledge and his critical approach was misinterpreted as aloofness. Griff, weighed down by his new responsibilities, pined for the laboratory. He resented the time required to be a good administrator. He labored with decisions and worried for days over issues that Mort would have dispatched in seconds. Both men were dissipating energy in pursuits unsuited to their strengths. Griff saw it clearly and resolved to remedy the situation. He waged a campaign to become Director of the Clinical Center. It was apparent to all that this job was associated with a level of stress incompatible with his accelerating angina. "No matter," he said, and carried the campaign forward. When, at last, the job was offered, the strategy became clear. He said, to paraphrase, "I can undertake this job only if you will bring Mort Lipsett back to assist me." After much negotiation, Mort did come back, but as Director of the Clinical Center. Griff, in his zeal to bring Mort "home," became the Associate Director. It was an important act of magnanimity: the two men provided the Clinical Center and the NIH with many years of inspired leadership, leadership uncommon in government service.

Mort and Griff died within months of each other. Both died of malignancy. Mort discovered a cerebellar tumor when he was unable to make a certain tennis shot that had been routine in the past. He ordered a CT scan and found the lesion. Griff had prostate cancer diagnosed as an incidental finding on the biopsy material from a TURP. Both men dealt nobly with their illness. Mort never discussed it except to acknowledge the problem and to let you know he was fine and "let's get on to substantive issues." Griff talked about his illness at length, never in a maudlin way, but in a clinical and analytical fashion.

Two events from this period stand out in memory. The first occurred when it became clear that Griff was failing. A Festschrift at the NIH was planned in his honor. Mort was to be the main speaker. He was receiving chemotherapy at the time and, at the last minute, decided he was too unwell to attend. I was summoned to his bedside and he handed me a handwritten speech and asked if I would read it in his stead. I said I would. He then asked if I would read it once in his presence. The opening line went something like this:

"It is a great pleasure to have the opportunity to speak on this occasion honoring Griff Ross, my best friend of more than 20 yr." I was struck by the line. This level of intimacy was not characteristic of Mort. After I had read the speech through, I got up to go and give the address. As I turned to leave, Mort said "Lynn, you won't forget the 'best friend' part, will you?" In retrospect, I believe that Mort did not trust himself to include the "best," the very concept he most wished, on that occasion, to convey. He thought it safer in my hands.

The second event happened over the phone. Griff was dying, it was said, and I called his hospital room in Texas for what I thought would be a last brief goodby. The first thing he told me was that he had four of the major things that kill people: heart disease, high blood pressure, an aneurism of a cerebral artery, and cancer. Otherwise, however, he was "doing fine!" Then, he launched into a discussion of his latest observations on gynecomastia, a side-effect of one of his medications. It was just like old times. He died 2 days later.

Different as these two men were, they were alike in fundamentally important ways. Both loved medicine and respected science. Both recognized the difference between scholarship and science and understood the sustaining force of science for medicine. Both loved the NIH and the ethos of those that worked there. Both loved young people and were comfortable in their presence. Both measured the worth of their careers by the accomplishments of their fellows. Both accepted as a first premise the orchestration of life by molecular messengers. Both found their greatest joy in the discovery of new truths.

The workplace created by Mort and Griff is unlikely ever to be recreated. The remarkable success of their trainees has been ascribed to the liberal funding of the intramural NIH, the high quality of the trainee "substrate" pool, and the research opportunities afforded by the newly developed technique of RIA. I believe that the most important factor was the unique complement of the personalities and strengths of these two men and their genuine friendship and mutual respect. This created an environment with few weaknesses. Between the poles of these two great personalities was a place for almost any combination of character and talent. Aspiration to greatness was encouraged and its germination carefully nurtured. When realized, it was never resented nor envied. Those of us that were the beneficiaries of this extraordinary "beginning" still count our blessings.

D. Lynn Loriaux
Division of Endocrinology
Oregon Health Sciences University
Portland, Oregon

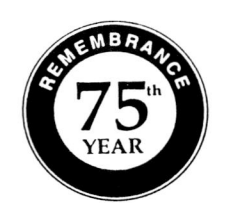

Remembrance: Leslie L. Iversen, Merck Sharp & Dohme Research Laboratories, Neuroscience Research Centre, Harlow, England. "The Axelrod Lab, 1964–1965"

I was lucky enough to spend a year working in Julie Axelrod's laboratory as a visiting postdoc 1964–1965. At that time I had recently completed Ph.D. studies at the University of Cambridge in England, on the topic of noradrenaline uptake sites in peripheral sympathetic nerves. I was supervised in Cambridge by Gordon Whitby, who had recently returned from working in Julie's lab where with Georg Hertting the phenomenon of catecholamine uptake as a means of inactivating and recycling catecholamines after their release from nerve terminals had just been discovered (1961).

The year at the National Institutes of Health working with Julie proved to be an extraordinarily intense experience. The NIH was still a young organization and very much in its heyday. At the time many of the best and brightest young U.S. physicians were attracted to work there for their military service—as an alternative to the battlefield in Indo-China. The whole place hummed with intellectual vigor and excitement, and to an Englishman who had been taught to make do with slender lab resources, the availability of almost unlimited support and facilities for medical research was heady stuff. Julie's lab was also in a period of high productivity—having already made very important advances in the late 1950s and early 1960s which lead to a more complete understanding of the metabolic pathways and disposition of catecholamines in the body. Particularly important were the discoveries of the *O*-methylation pathway for catecholamine metabolism, and the role of uptake as an inactivation mechanism.

In Julie's lab I was able to pursue further work on catecholamine uptake in peripheral tissues, and also by collaborating with a French visitor to the lab, Jacques Glowinski, to explore the uptake and metabolism of catecholamines in brain. Jacques and Julie had seen that the unique ability of adrenergic neurones to accumulate radiolabeled noradrenaline and dopamine made it possible to use these radiochemicals to study the disposition and turnover of the neuronal pool of catecholamines in brain, even though these neurons represented only a small fraction of the total population in most brain areas. The collaboration with Jacques Glowinski came to be the major focus of my work during that year. As with everyone else in the small group working in his lab at that time, Julie displayed an intense interest in what we were doing—and produced a constant stream of ideas for us to pursue: far more ideas than was humanly possible to act upon! Indeed Jacques and I would wait with some apprehension for Julie to return to the lab after his customary foray into the library after lunch each day. He would invariably have read and been excited by some new discovery—and would have seen how it might impact on our own research programs. Julie has displayed throughout his career a remarkable vein of creativity, a rare and precious human commodity. During my time in the lab Julie also remained very active in the laboratory—undertaking experiments almost every day (mainly on pineal melatonin metabolism at that time). He would wait by the scintillation counter with intense excitement for the day's results to be printed out. So impatient was he to learn the result, he would often turn the machine to print out at 0.1-min intervals in order to see whether the experiment had worked or not!

The year itself was a very important experience for me, but it also proved to have far-reaching consequences for the remainder of my career. At the time I met several people with whom close professional and personal friendships developed—these included Jacques Glowinski, Sol Snyder, Irv Kopin, Arnie Eisenfeld, Jose Musacchio, Seymour Kety, Lou Sokoloff, and Dick Wurtman. After leaving the lab I came to know others who joined later and several of these too became close colleagues and friends—including Ira Black (who came to work with me in Cambridge after having been in Julie's lab), Hans Thoenen, Perry Molinoff, Joe Coyle, Terry Resine, and Mike Brownstein.

Julie was responsible for training a remarkably talented group of scientists in what was then the modern biochemical approach to pharmacology—which came to dominate in the 1960s and 1970s. His personal committment and enthusiasm for science helped to inspire many of us with our own longstanding belief that research was the right career for us. We all owe him a considerable debt, and look forward to celebrating with him later this year his 80th birthday.

Les Iversen
Merck Sharp & Dohme Research Laboratories
Neuroscience Research Centre
Harlow, England

Received February 18, 1992.
"Remembrance" articles discuss people and events as remembered by the author. The opinion(s) expressed are solely those of the writer and do not reflect the view of the Journal or The Endocrine Society.

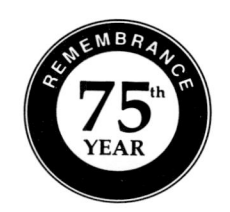

The Concept of Negative Feedback—Moore and Price

I met Drs. Carl R. Moore and Dorothy Price when I began my Ph.D. work under Dr. Moore in 1948 at the University of Chicago. Carl Moore was chairman of the zoology department at that time. He did not have a personal secretary and his office was always open to anyone knocking on his door. To the knock he would answer in his big voice, "Come In." He was a tall, blond, outgoing man who sat behind his large roll-top desk. There was a microscope on a table behind him and a typewriter on a table next to the desk. The room was blue with pipe smoke. Dorothy Price was rather slender with graying hair and at that time she was an assistant professor. Dorothy was well liked by the graduate students, especially those with whom she taught in the laboratories of the division of biological sciences sequence. She obviously had the students' interests at heart.

For most of their research lives these two people had been trying to determine the mechanisms involved in sex differentiation in mammals. The driving force for Moore was the description by Frank Lillie of the freemartin. The freemartin is the intersex female cotwin of male-female twinning in cattle. (Freemartins may also occur in such twinning in other two-toed ungulates.) Lillie's hypothesis was that the male cotwin produced a hormone from the testis which inhibited the development of the reproductive tract of the female cotwin. Moore began a series of experiments to understand the processes of sex development after finishing his doctoral thesis on fertilization and parthenogenesis of sea urchin eggs. The freemartin hypothesis of Lillie had led others to the idea that the female sex hormones had antagonistic effects on male reproductive tracts and testes and that male hormones had antagonistic effects on ovaries and uteri. In the absence of pure steroid hormones this idea was very popular, especially in Europe. To get pure preparations of androgens, Carl Moore and his research assistant, Dorothy Price, were working on a mammalian assay for androgens with F. C. Koch and his associates in the biochemistry department. They hoped to use the pure androgens to help understand the freemartin.

The study of the freemartin was postponed by the hypotheses about sex hormone antagonism. Moore was very skeptical about male and female hormone antagonism. He designed experiments to determine the effects of the male and female hormones on both sexes of rats. The hormones injected were impure extracts: bull testis extract for androgen, estrin from human placentae (prepared by Gustavson and D'Armour) for estrogen, and pregnancy urine and pituitary implants for gonadotropins. Young adult and mature adult rats, both normal and castrate, were used. (Most of the initial experiments were on males with some observations on females.). The effects of the injections were: 1) estrin did not cause a change in the accessory glands of castrate rats, nor did testis extract change the uterus of spayed rats; 2) injection of estrin in normal males caused a reduction of testis weight and also decreased the weight of the accessory glands; 3) injection of testis extract in normal females caused cessation of estrous cycles; 4) injection of testis extract in males caused cessation of spermatogenesis and decreased testis weight, but the accessory glands remained enlarged; and 5) injection of estrin in females enlarged the uterus, but the animals stopped cycling. Injection of each preparation with gonadotropic substances either completely or partially reversed the effects of the steroid hormone treatments. Both investigators were very puzzled by the results, but the answer was supplied by Dorothy Price, who realized that the steroid extracts were inhibiting the secretion of the gonadotropic stimulating hormones from the pituitary. In their papers (1, 2), Moore and Price concluded "a substance the hypophysis could not supply" was absent when the steroid extracts were used, and this substance was supplied when the gonadotropic preparations were injected into rats treated with the steroid extracts. Moore presented the work in a paper in London in 1930, and both authors quickly published the results in a short paper (1) and a long one later (2). Thus, by 1932 the major hypothesis and its evidence had been presented. It was not modified during their lifetimes by either Carl Moore or Dorothy Price because, except for a few additional studies on females by Moore's students, they did little further work on the negative feedback theory.

Moore and Price felt that they could explain cycling in female rats and testicular responses in male rats on the basis of their hypothesis. They knew that light could trigger gonadal activity in some annually breeding mammals and birds and felt that the cessation of breeding activity in these species was due to the feedback of the gonadal steroid hormones. However, Moore remained interested in species that bred annually. He found negative feedback a possible explanation for the cessation of breeding activity in annual breeding mammals that were not light sensitive (13-lined ground squirrels and prairie dogs) but felt that the long quiescence of the reproductive system made negative feedback a difficult explanation for these species.

Moore and Price were familiar with the work of D. Roy McCullagh (3) who with his brother Perry hypothesized a nonsteroidal feedback mechanism to the pituitary. Moore tried some experiments but could get a clear-cut effect that he could ascribe to inhibin. Real evidence became available after new techniques of tissue culture of granulosa cells were developed (4). Perry McCullagh was a secretary of the American Association for the Study of Internal Secretions (now The Endocrine

---

Received February 25, 1992.

"Remembrance" articles discuss people and events as remembered by the author. The opinion(s) expressed are solely those of the writer and do not reflect the view of the Journal of The Endocrine Society.

Society) in 1938 and president of The Endocrine Society in 1958. I talked to him once about a Cleveland Sigma Xi event over the telephone, and he was surprised that anyone remembered either him or his work on inhibin. Although Moore and Price did know about inhibin they did not know the work of Holweg and Junkmann (5) in Germany. Price later said it was a more limited and less international climate for science at that time and, of course, there was a worldwide depression. The real understanding of the research of Holweg and Junkmann came with the publication by Harris in 1955 of "The neural control of the pituitary gland" (6).

Carl Moore was raised in the Missouri Ozarks and loved the outdoors. He was a fly fisherman and had a summer home on Elk Lake in Michigan, where he had a shed he used for his microscopic studies. His reputation was firmly established before the negative feedback theory was published. He had already shown that scrota of mammals maintained testicular temperatures below body temperatures and thereby prevented heat damage to spermatogenic tubules. His experiments included wrapping the scrota of rams in flannel pajamas made by his wife (the rams grazed on Chicago's Midway) and heating only part of the scrotum of guinea pigs to 37 C. In 1950, he received an award from the American Urological Association in recognition of his studies of cryptorchidism and the function of the scrotum.

After the publication of the negative feedback papers Moore returned to his first love, the analysis of the factors involved in sexual differentiation in the embryo with sidetracks to other problems in reproduction (*e.g.* effects of high altitude, role of the ovarian germinal epithelium). One of these side-tracks involved him in a court case in 1938. His students had found that estrogens (they used face creams) were absorbed through the skin of rodents and that they had systemic effects on uterine and mammary growth even in male guinea pigs. This work was first reported in *JAMA*, and that journal's editor, Morris Fishbein, wrote an editorial about the uncontrolled use of steroids by the cosmetic industry. About 24 h after this editorial was printed, the AMA, Fishbein, Moore, and the graduate students were all sued by the cosmetic industry. The suit ended in a draw because no human studies were done, even though steroid activity was expressed in terms of rat assays as claimed by the defense. The estrogenic face creams remained on the market. By the late 1930s Moore was using the oppossum for his studies because it was born before the gonads and reproductive ducts had differentiated and the young could be castrated in the pouch with less damage than treating the fetuses of pregnant rats. Moore's work brought Dr. Alfred Jost (see Ref. 7) to Chicago in 1949 to present his experiments on rabbit embryos. Moore was very pleased with Jost's work and was able to get him to visit the class on the Biology of Sex to explain his experiments. In 1950 Moore went to Paris and reported on his oppossum studies at a colloquium. This was his last major conference, as illness was beginning to take its toll.

Moore was president of the American Association for the Study of Internal Secretions from 1944–1946 during World War II and in 1955 was awarded the first Endocrine Society Medal and Certificate of Award. He was a member of the National Academy of Science and active in the National Research Council as a member of the Committee for Research on the Problems of Sex, the Committee on Human Reproduction, and the Committee on Growth. He supported strongly the research of Kinsey on male and female reproductive behavior against the attacks of clergymen and others. He believed that research alone would lead to the understanding of the biological and psychological aspects of sexual activity. Carl Moore died of cancer in the fall of 1955 at the age of 63. He had been chairman of zoology at Chicago since 1934. Moore was devoted to teaching and considered it a proper obligation and privilege to be able to teach students. The different research projects and the numerous awards presented to Moore have been described by Price (8).

Dorothy Price was raised in Illinois. She started her graduate work in 1922 at Chicago, but family finances forced her to seek employment. She was a first a research assistant for Lillie and later a research associate for Moore. She finished her doctoral work in 1935 on the development of the prostate and its responses to androgens (9). She used the newly isolated androgens from Koch's laboratory for some of these studies. She was hired as an assistant professor by the zoology department in the 1947. She was, I believe, the only woman on a natural science faculty of any major research university at that time. After her doctoral studies, Dorothy Price also turned to the study of sex differentiation. Her approach was to use organ culture of embryonic male and female reproductive tracts with and without their associated gonads or with gonads of the opposite sex. She published numerous papers on the results of these studies with Drs. Evelina Ortiz and Johanna Zaaijer in what she described as a "long-term, long-distance collaboration between Chicago, Leiden, and Puerto Rico." She was promoted regularly and was a full professor well before she retired in 1967. Dorothy Price remained a lively and interesting person devoted to her science even after her retirement. She continued her studies using organ culture and wrote some historical discussions on the development of sex. She was appointed the Boerhaave Professor (an honorary visiting chair) at the University of Leiden in 1967 and was awarded their Medal for Distinguished Service that year as well. In later years, Dorothy described her role in the negative feedback hypothesis and how she thought that they had backed into the hypothesis in the process of studying sex hormone antagonism. She also discussed later developments with reference to the original hypothesis (10). We should remember that although our present knowledge is more complete, her insight gave the right explanation to the results obtained in 1930. Dorothy continued to work in Leiden after her retirement but also often came back to Chicago. In November 1980, I received notice from Drs. Ortiz and Zaaijer of Dorothy Price's death in Leiden on November 17. Women in endocrinology should consider Dorothy Price an appropriate ancestral role model because she brought talent, insight, patient experimentation, and steadfast courage to the science that interested her, in spite of the tremendous odds against the progress of women in science, even at so enlightened an institution as the

University of Chicago.

Darhl Foreman
Department of Biology
Case Western Reserve University

References

1. **Moore CR, Price D** 1930 The question of sex hormone antagonism. Proc Soc Exp Biol Med 28:38–40
2. **Moore CR, Price D** 1932 Gonad hormone functions and the reciprocal influence between gonads and hypophysis with its bearing on the problem of sex hormone antagonism. Am J Anat 50:13–67
3. **McCullagh DR** 1932 Dual endocrine activity of the testes. Science 76:19–20
4. **Schwartz NB** 1991 Why I was told not to study inhibin and what I did about it. Endocrinology 129:1690–1691
5. **Holweg W, Junkmann K** 1932 Die hormonal-nervose Regulierung der Funkion des Hypophysenborderlappens. Klin Wochenschr 11:321–323
6. **Harris GW** 1955 Neural control of the pituitary gland. Monographs of the Physiological Society. No. 3. Edward Arnold Ltd, London
7. Unité de Recherches sur l'Endocrinologie du Dévelopement INSERM 1991 Rememberance of Dr. Alfred Jost. Endocrinology 129:2274–2276
8. **Price D** 1974 Carl Richard Moore. Biographical memoirs. Proc Natl Acad Sci USA 45:385–412
9. **Price D** 1936 Normal development of the prostate and seminal vesicles of the rat with a study of experimental postnatal modifications. Am J Anat 60:79–126
10. **Price D** 1975 Feedback control of gonadal and hypophysial hormones. Evolution of the concept. In: Meites J, Donovan BT, McCann SM, (eds) Pioneers in Neuroendocrinology

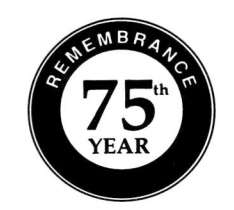

Thyroxine Transport and the Free Hormone Hypothesis

In 1952, while working with J. E. Rall and Rulon Rawson at the Memorial-Sloan Kettering Cancer Center in New York, our attention was focused on thyroid cancer, and we became interested in the nature of iodine compounds in blood that might have their origin in the tumor. At that time, it was known that the circulating thyroid hormone, T_4, contrary to that found in the thyroid gland, was reversibly bound to plasma protein. Efforts to characterize the binding protein, or proteins, were under way when a paper appeared from Mill Hill by Gordon *et al.* (1) that suddenly clarified the issue. They had applied the new technique of zone electrophoresis on filter paper which permitted sampling of the separated proteins for ^{131}I-labeled hormone, and they showed that most of the radioactive iodine was sharply localized between the α_1 and α_2 globulins. Henry Kunkel of the Rockefeller Institute had just published an elegant paper with Arne Tiselius (2) describing how proteins migrate through the erratic capillary spaces of the filter paper, and, since my laboratory was across the road, I paid him a visit to find out how it was done. He advised me to procure two pieces of plate glass, two battery jars on which to suspend them, two telephone batteries which I was to break open for their carbon electrodes, and a power supply. I used a battery pack obtained from Mones Berman and, with this simple apparatus, quickly confirmed the finding of Gordon *et al.* that thyroxine was, indeed, attached to a minor plasma protein (3), named thyroxine binding protein (then thyroxine binding globulin or TBG). We resisted the temptation to call the protein transthyrin, but a short time later, a very similar protein that carries corticosteroid, which is now known to belong to the same gene family (4, 5), was named transcortin (6). Still later, we helped the committee on nomenclature of the International Union of Biochemistry to rename a second T_4-transport protein known as thyroxine binding prealbumin. The name transthyretin was chosen to reflect its additional role in transporting retinol through interaction with retinol binding protein.

Although the crude electrophoretic apparatus provided excellent protein separation, the amount of T_4 associated with TBG increased continuously with increasing T_4 concentration (7). A simple technical modification we made after moving to the NIH in 1954, which we termed reverse-flow electrophoresis (8), avoided the inclusion of albumin-bound T_4 in the TBG zone. Only then could we accurately measure the T_4-binding capacity of TBG, especially when the TBG concentration was low. This allowed us to investigate the clinical enigma of an apparent euthyroid state in nephrosis, where the protein-bound iodine was in the hypothyroid range (9), and in pregnancy, where the protein-bound iodine was in the hyperthyroid range (10). We found that the TBG capacity for T_4 was low in nephrosis (11) and high in pregnancy (12). A few other workers were on the same track. Dowling *et al.* (13) also described the increased TBG in pregnancy and later attributed this to the effect of increased estrogen (14). Several years earlier, Recant and Riggs (15) had suggested that the low protein binding of T_4 in nephrosis could explain the euthyroid state in the face of a low T_4 concentration if an increase in the free hormone fraction occurred and if the free hormone entered the tissues at a normal rate. This was the birth of the free hormone hypothesis.

In 1956, Ed Rall and I were invited to report our work at the Laurentian Hormone Conference at Mount Tremblant, Quebec, Canada. We then made the first attempt to quantify the free hormone concentration in blood by an indirect calculation based on renal clearance (16). We also calculated the value from first principles, knowing the association constants of the major binding proteins (16–18). When Ken Sterling, Jack Oppenheimer, Sid Ingbar, and their respective colleagues were able to measure free T_4 (see Ref. 18), our conclusions proved to be correct not only qualitatively but even quantitatively.

The free hormone hypothesis—which proposed that the rate at which thyroxine is metabolized, and the hormonal effect of T_4, are directly proportional to the free or unbound thyroxine concentration in plasma—has become a central feature of thyroid physiology, and the measurement of free T_4 is now a mainstay of clinical thyroidology. However, it is not free of controversy. Even now (19, 20) investigators continue to attempt to understand why a specific trace protein has been recruited to transport T_4 from the thyroid glad to the periphery. As we said at the Laurentian Hormone Conference in 1957, this is basically a philosophical question to which we, perhaps, will never have a satisfying answer. Nevertheless, we have over the years had the truly satisfying experience of working on the chemistry of the transport proteins with Harold Edelhoch, Hans Cahnmann, and our younger colleagues (21). We also had the pleasure of seeing Colin Blake and colleagues' data on the high resolution structure of the transthyretin molecule (*c.f.* 20) and more recently, learning about the genetic aberrations of TBG, with Sam Refetoff finding the mutations one by one (22), about other proteins in the TBG gene family (4, 20), and about transthyretin variants and the biosynthesis of transthyretin in the choroid plexus (20). T_4 transport proteins and the free

---

Received February 24, 1992.

"Remembrance" articles discuss people and events as remembered by the author. The opinion(s) expressed are solely those of the writer and do not reflect the view of the Journal or The Endocrine Society.

thyroxine hypothesis persist as fascinating models for the passage of small molecules and their transporters through the circulation, past the capillary walls, and into cells.

Jacob Robbins
National Institute of Diabetes
and Digestive and Kidney Diseases
National Institutes of Health

References

1. **Gordon AH, Gross J, O'Connor D, Pitt-Rivers R** 1952 Nature of the circulating thyroid hormone-plasma protein complex. Nature 169:19–20
2. **Kunkel HG, Tiselius A** 1951 Electrophoresis of proteins on filter paper. J Gen Physiol 35:89–118
3. **Robbins J, Rall JE** 1952 Zone electrophoresis in filter paper of serum I-131 after radioiodide administration. Proc Soc Expt Biol Med 81:530–536
4. **Flink IL, Bailey TJ, Gustefson A, Markham BE, Morkin E** 1986 Complete amino acid sequence of human thyroxine-binding globulin deduced from cloned DNA: close homology to the serum antiproteases. Proc Natl Acad Sci USA 83:7708–7712
5. **Hammond GL, Smith CL, Goping IS, Underhill DA, Harley MJ, Raventor J, Musto NA, Gunsalus GL, Bardin CW** 1987 Primary structure of human corticosteroid binding globulin deduced from hepatic and pulmonary cDNAs, exhibits homology with serine protese inhibitors. Proc Natl Acad Sci USA 84:5153–5157
6. **Slaunwhite Jr WR, Sandberg AA** 1959 Transcortin: a corticosteroid-binding protein of plasma. J Clin Invest 38:384–391
7. **Robbins J, Rall JE** 1955 Thyroxine binding capacity of serum in normal man. J Clin Invest 34:1324–1330
8. **Robbins J** 1956 Reverse flow electrophoresis: a method for determining the thyroxine-binding capacity of serum protein. Arch Biochem Biophys 63:461–469
9. **Heinemann J, Johnson CE, Man EB** 1948 Serum precipitable iodine concentrations during pregnancy. J Clin Invest 27:91–97
10. **Peters JP, Man EB** 1948 The relation of albumin to precipitable iodine of serum. J Clin Invest 27:397–405
11. **Robbins J, Rall JE, Petermann ML** 1957 Thyroxine binding by serum and urine proteins in nephrosis: qualitative aspects. J Clin Invest 36:1333–1342
12. **Robbins J, Nelson JH** 1958 Thyroxine binding by serum protein in pregnancy and in the newborn. J Clin Invest 37:153–159
13. **Dowling JT, Freinkel N, Ingbar SH** 1956 Thyroxine binding by sera of pregnant women, newborn infants and women with spontaneous abortion. J Clin Invest 35:1263–1276
14. **Dowling JT, Freinkel N, Ingbar SH** 1956 Effect of diethylstilbestrol on the binding of thyroxine in serum. J Clin Endocrinol Metab 16:1491–1506
15. **Recant L, Riggs DS** 1952 Thyroid function in nephrosis. J Clin Invest 31:789–797
16. **Robbins J, Rall JE** 1957 The interaction of thyroid hormones and protein in biological fluids. Recent Prog Horm Res 13:161–202
17. **Robbins J, Rall JE** 1960 Proteins associated with the thyroid hormones. Physiol Rev 40:415–489
18. **Robbins J, Rall JE** 1967 The iodine-containing hormones. In: Gray CH, Bacharach AL (eds) Hormones in Blood, ed 2. Academic Press, London, pp 383–490
19. **Mendel CM** 1989 The free hormone hypothesis: a physiologically based mathematical model. Endocr Rev 10:232–274
20. **Robbins J** 1991 Thyroid hormone transport proteins and the physiology of hormone binding. In Braverman LE, Utiger RD (eds) The Thyroid, ed 6. JB Lippincott, Philadelphia, pp 111–125
21. **Robbins J, Cheng SY, Gershengorn MD, Glinoer D, Cahnmann HJ, Edelhoch H** 1978 Thyroxine transport proteins of plasma: molecular properties and biosynthesis. Recent Prog Horm Res 34:477–519
22. **Refetoff S** 1989 Inherited thyroxine-binding globulin abnormalities in man. Endocr Rev 10:275–293

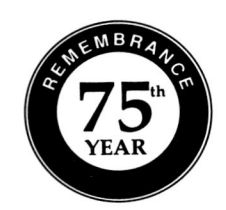

Remembrance: Columbia University's Endocrine Journal Club

Without exaggeration, New Yorkers may claim that the Columbia Endocrine Journal Club has had an important influence on endocrine scholarship in the New York City area over a period of nearly 40 yr. Started in 1953, the Journal Club continues until the present, albeit now under new auspices.[1] Examining the list of names of some of the endocrinologists who have participated in this activity suggest that this influence has spread to many parts of the country and indeed to other countries as well. Since many of the people who attended these weekly sessions were at the beginning of their careers, it may be presumed that these meetings played a helpful role in their development as endocrinologists.

During the years since 1953, when the late Dr. Joseph W. Jailer and I initiated this Journal Club, at Columbia's College of Physicians and Surgeons, its format was changed several times. The most successful arrangement, however, lasted more than a quarter of a century. Obviously the Journal Club persisted because many people found it worth their while to attend. Over the years there were always about 50 people in the various institutions of higher learning in the metropolitan area, who were interested enough in current developments in those areas of endocrinology we dealt with to trek up to 168th Street, in Washington Heights. They came to this out-of-the way site of the College of P&S from all parts of the City and even from other cities, e.g. New Haven, Newark, and Philadelphia.

For many, this was a weekly routine; the Journal Club met every week on Tuesday evening. This invariant schedule continued for about 30 weeks of the academic year and gave assurance to those people who were interested in attending that our sessions would begin every Tuesday at 5:30 pm and end at 7:00 pm. Only a heavy snow storm would induce us to postpone the meeting. Those who came from afar could be assured that a program addressing various subjects had been arranged for them and that 10–25 like-minded people would be present to join in the ensuing discussions. The durability of the enterprise was due in large measure to this unwavering schedule.

Another characteristic of the Journal Club that was, and is still, critical for its longevity was that each meeting inevitably turned out to be a social event. Not only was it an educational experience, attendance was an enjoyment. In many cases, the participants (there were no members, anyone was welcome) already knew each other, or else soon got to know each other and thus the Journal Club became a weekly reunion of old and new friends. It takes no effort whatever to make a gathering pleasurable when the participants are congenial, have shared experiences and common professional interests, and convene at a noncompetitive occasion. In addition, to sweeten the proceedings still further, a banquet of Chinese food was often arranged for to round out the evening. Several times a year the banquet was catered at either one of the conference rooms at P&S or at one of New York's wonderful Chinese restaurants. I still remember one dinner where the piece de resistance was a gorgeous roast suckling pig.

The usual format of each weekly meeting consisted of 10–20 min oral descriptions of three to five recently published papers, each given by a different analyst. The emphasis in each case was on analysis. Because of its usual pejorative connotation, the word, criticism, is less appropriate. The speakers and the papers to be presented were selected by a small group of elders who met a half hour before each session to prepare the program for subsequent meetings. In making assignments the experience of each speaker was taken into account. Special effort was made to provide less experienced presenters with practice even when such a choice may have afforded a less than perfect analysis. Not surprisingly, the Journal Club played an important role by providing a friendly forum where budding, and frequently even mature scientists, could sharpen their communicative, polemic, and ratiocinative skills. Impressive improvement in these skills was achieved by many people, even by some who began with no obvious talent. The chief element in that improvement was having the opportunity to practice before a tolerant audience and receiving appropriate sympathetic suggestions. For those who served as mentors, the process was especially satisfying.

It is my judgment that the benefit the participants received from their attendance went beyond the acquisition of the facts of endocrinology. Of course they learned many facts but even 30–40 yr ago the science consisted of so many subspecialities, each of which had its own inherent complexities, that it was unreasonable to use the technique of weekly seminars to bring attention to the current developments in

---

Received February 27, 1992.

'Remembrance' articles discuss people and events as remembered by the author. The opinion(s) expressed are solely those of the writer and do not reflect the view of the Journal or The Endocrine Society.

[1] Six years ago, the Journal Club was moved to the Rockefeller University where, under the mentorship of Drs. H. L. Bradlow, M. Levitz, and C. Monder, it still thrives. At its meeting on February 4, 1992, there were 32 attendees.

all the facets of the discipline. Moreover, since we did not have the expertise to consider every branch of the subject, some areas of endocrine research were deliberately neglected. The subjects we concentrated on were: the biochemistry of the steroids and related pituitary hormones and the physiological and pathophysiological aspects of the adrenals, testes, ovaries, placenta, and pituitary. Since our attendees consisted of MDs and PhDs, our programs were constructed so as to provide items of interest to each group at every session. While imparting endocrine facts was an important pedagogical objective of each presentation, it was not the most important. Participants benefited most from observing how experienced practitioners analyze scientific papers. Because the presenters were usually expert in the subject they discussed, their analytic technique, as well as their expository competence, provided the auditors the greatest educational value.

Thus the longevity of the Journal Club was due to these several reasons. This format for teaching scientific scholarship is very effective, teaching scientific facts is easier; teaching scientific creativity is more difficult, perhaps impossible. Needless to say, the free-wheeling discussion that followed each talk contributed significantly to the further education of young students as well as aging professors.

Reminiscing may be one of the few pleasurable pastimes left to the aged, at least to those whose memory is unimpaired. Reminiscing about the Journal Club has again brought me much pleasure, it could not be otherwise, for the rewards of this experience, shared over so many years with people of such quality, busying ourselves with the analysis of a subject of such fascination was, not surprisingly, one of the delights of my life.

Following is a list of the names of some of the endocrinologists who attended the Columbia Endocrine Journal Club at one time or another. Obviously many more people than those identified below participated in the 1000 or so sessions held over the past 4 decades but since attendance was not recorded and since no one's memory is perfect, the names of many are, unhappily, omitted. Among those listed below are the nationals of 18 different countries. By now, as many as 90 of those listed have attained the rank of Professor (of endocrinology or one of its related disciplines). Eleven were elected members of the Council of The Endocrine Society and of these 5 became President. There have been many prize winners; the latest is Assistant Professor Synthia Mellon who in 1991 received the Richard E. Weitzman Memorial Award of The Endocrine Society. The participants (1953–____) are: C. A. Abrams, D. H. Albert, N. G. Anderson, M. Arcos, L. Bandy, D. S. Bartosik, E. E. Baulieu, F. J. Bell, S. Bernstein, V. Black, J. A. Blaquier, T. Bledsoe, S. L. Blethen, J. Bogumil, E. Bolte, A. M. Bongiovanni, H. L. Bradlow, J. A. Brasel, J. Brind, S. Burstein, J. J. Byrne, H. I. Calvin, R. E. Canfield, D. I. Cargill, A. Chapdelaine, F. I. Chasalow, C.-L. C. Chen, N. P. Christy, G. Concolino, C. Corporchet, F. S. Cowchock, R. R. David, W. R. Dixon, N. M. Drayer, W. D. Drucker, I. Dyrenfurth, W. Eberlein, I. S. Edelman, B. F. Erlanger, M. Feigelson, P. Feigelson, M. Feldman, M. Ferin, T. H. Finlay, J. Fishman, S. Franklin, A. G. Frantz, D. K. Fukushima, T. F. Gallagher, H. M. Gandy, F. J. Gasparini, J. J. Gold, D. S. Goodman, E. Gurpide, R. W. Harrison, W. C. Hembree, W. L. Hermann, R. B. Hershcopf, R. B. Hochberg, V. P. Hollander, R. M. Hoyte, G. M. Jacobsohn, G. M. Jagiello, J. W. Jailer, R. Jewelewicz, S. Kammerman, S. L. Kaplan, M. S. Khan, J. I. Kitay, D. L. Kleinberg, S. G. Korenman, A. I. Knowlton, S. Ladany, J. H. Laragh, W. J. LeMaire, M. Levitz, S. Lieberman, V. Lipmann, M. E. Lippman, M. Lipsett, J. N. Loeb, V. Luine, B. M. Luttrell, P. C. MacDonald, P. D. McDonald, K. O. Martin, L. Martini, C. P. Martucci, S. Mellon, G. R. Merriam, H. Mickan, L. Miller, W. L. Miller, M. E. Monaco, C. Monder, F. Naftolin, M. I. New, J. H. Oppenheimer, L. Ponticorvo, V. V. K. Prasad, J. Raus, H. Rifkin, P. Robel, J. L. Roberts, K. D. Roberts, M. S. Roginsky, R. S. Rosenfeld, W. Rosner, K. J. Ryan, H. A. Salhanick, A. A. Sandberg, E. Sandberg, W. H. Sawyer, F. Schatz, J. F. Schwers, J. E. Sealey, S. J. Segal, M. R. Sherman, P. K. Siiteri, S. Solomon, S. S. Solomon, K. Sterling, J. J. Stevens, M. I. Surks, O. Tanizawa, S. Teich, L. Tseng, S. Ulick, T. Usui, R. L. VandeWiele, T. VandeHoeven, E. Z. Wallace, P. Warne, M. Warren, G. Weiss, A. J. Wolfson, R. S. Yalow, P. E. Zimmering, B. Zumoff, U. Zor.

Seymour Lieberman[2]
St. Lukes-Roosevelt Institute for Health Sciences
New York, New York

---

[2] Present address: The St. Luke's-Roosevelt Institute for Health Sciences, 432 West 58 Street, New York, New York 10019.

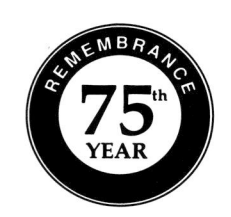

Remembrance: The Discovery of the Hypothalamic Gonadotropin-Releasing Hormone Pulse Generator and of its Physiological Significance

Shortly after a specific RIA for monkey LH became available in the late 1960s, we began to investigate the dynamics of its secretion in a variety of physiological and experimental circumstances. One such early study was designed to determine whether a circadian rhythm in the plasma levels of the peptide could be detected. To this end, hourly blood samples were obtained for 24 h from chronically ovariectomized monkeys restrained in primate chairs. We were surprised to find frequent, apparently random, and often large LH peaks during this period that were unrelated to the time of day or to perturbations in the environment (1). Similarly unstable LH concentrations had been reported previously in gonadectomized rats (2) sampled at 1-h intervals or longer. Having thoroughly reassured ourselves that the instability of our hormone measurements in the monkey were not attributable to assay error, a major concern at the time, we proceeded to take a much closer look at this apparent secretory discontinuity by sampling blood every 10, 20, or 30 min. These experiments were performed in ovariectomized monkeys chronically fitted with indwelling cardiac catheters and restrained in primate chairs. The results were literally breathtaking. We observed strikingly large, rhythmic oscillations in plasma LH concentrations with a period of approximately 1 h, leading us to coin the term "circhoral" (about 1 h) to describe this phenomenon (3). The peptide levels rose from nadir to maximum in a single sampling period (10 or 20 min) and then declined exponentially at a rate approximating that of exogenous rhesus monkey LH for the remainder of the hour. These observations suggested that the oscillatory pattern of LH seen in the peripheral circulation must be the consequence of brief intermittent releases of LH from the pituitary gland, and that the "major portion of the elevated mean LH levels in ovariectomized animals can be accounted for by these pulsatile discharges" (3). More importantly, we concluded that "... these discharges may be due to intermittent signals from the central nervous system ... which, in turn, result in an increased production of LH-releasing factor ..." (3).

We recently discovered that a group of French investigators, also studying the diurnal variations of plasma gonadotropin levels in men and women reported, in 1970, (4) an unambiguous rhythmic pulsatile LH pattern with a period of 3–4 h in some of their subjects and were led to the conclusion that this rhythm was of physiological rather than experimental origin. Unfortunately, these workers did not, to my knowledge, pursue their observations and their paper, published contemporaneously with ours in the rhesus monkey, remained unknown to us until now.

In any case, these rhythmic pulsatile patterns of LH secretion were described soon thereafter in a large number of vertebrate species, their origin in the rhythmic discharge of GnRH into the pituitary portal circulation was confirmed, and the putative neuronal construct responsible for this phenomenon was localized to the region of the arcuate nucleus in the mediobasal hypothalamus (see Ref. 5 for review).

But the striking rhythmic patterns of pulsatile LH secretion remained in the realm of pure phenomenology for some 8 yr after their discovery. The physiological significance of intermittent LH secretion did not become evident until attempts were made to restore gonadotropin secretion in rhesus monkeys in whom endogenous GnRH secretion was abolished by lesions in the mediobasal hypothalamus. Continuous infusion of GnRH into such animals, while initially stimulating LH release for a day or so, failed to sustain LH secretion, the gonadotropin returning to undetectable levels despite continued administration of the decapeptide (5). Replacement with intermittent GnRH administration, however, at the frequency of one pulse per hour (the physiological frequency of LH pulses) did restore continued secretion of LH and FSH to prelesion levels (6). Furthermore, shifting from pulsatile to continuous administration of GnRH led to a decline in gonadotropin levels to zero, the consequence of a desensitization of the gonadotropes (7). These and related findings in the rhesus monkey led to the conclusion that the intermittency of the GnRH signal, within a relatively narrow window of frequencies, is an obligatory component of the neuroendocrine control system that governs normal gonadotropin secretion. These fundamental physiological observations in a nonhuman primate were transferred with remarkable rapidity to the clinical arena in the treatment of infertility attributable to hypothalamic dysfunction and in the suppression of inappropriate gonadotropin secretion (*e.g.* precocious puberty).

Received February 27, 1992.

"Remembrance" articles discuss people and events as remembered by the author. The opinion(s) expressed are solely those of the writer and do not reflect the view of the Journal or The Endocrine Society.

REMEMBRANCE

Ernst Knobil
H. Wayne Hightower Professor in the Medical Sciences
The University of Texas Medical School at Houston

References

1. **Atkinson LE, Bhattacharya AN, Monroe SE, Dierschke DJ, Knobil E** 1970 Effects of gonadectomy on plasma LH concentrations in the rhesus monkey. Endocrinology 87:847–849
2. **Gay VL, Midgley AR** 1969 Response of the adult rat to orchidectomy and ovariectomy as determined by LH radioimmunoassay. Endocrinology 84:1359–1364
3. **Dierschke DJ, Bhattacharya AN, Atkinson LE, Knobil E** 1970 Circhoral oscillations of plasma LH levels in the ovariectomized rhesus monkey. Endocrinology 87:850–853
4. **Dolais J, Valleron A-J, Grapin A-M, Rosselin G** 1970 Etude de l'hormone luteinisante humaine (HLH) au cours du nycthemere. C R Acad Sci [III] 270:3123–3126
5. **Knobil E** 1980 The neuroendocrine control of the menstrual cycle. Recent Prog Horm Res 36:53–88
6. **Nakai Y, Plant TM, Hess DL, Keogh EJ, Knobil E** 1978 On the sites of the negative and positive feedback actions of estradiol in the control of gonadotropin secretion in the rhesus monkey. Endocrinology 102:1008–1009
7. **Belchetz P, Plant TM, Nakai Y, Keogh EJ, Knobil E** 1978 Hypophysial responses to continuous and intermittent delivery of hypothalamic gonadotropin releasing hormone. Science 202:631–633

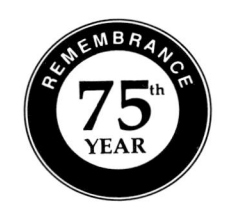

Remembrance: Calcitonin: Discovery and Early Development

In 1954, I was invited by Felix Bronner to present an evening lecture on calcium homeostasis at the first Gordon Conference on Bone and Teeth. Realizing how little was known of this important subject, I decided to make it my life work. The first step was find an accurate method of determining plasma calcium. I adapted the method of Fales (1), which depended on the titration of calcium with EDTA, using ammonium purpurate as indicator. The titration was plotted on graph paper and an eraser was used to permit reusing the paper. With this technique, we demonstrated the remarkable stability of plasma calcium in normal human subjects, and also observed the rapid recovery of normal plasma calcium levels in dogs within a few hours after infusion of calcium or EDTA.

Evidence for calcitonin was first obtained in our laboratory (2) in 1958. We were infusing dogs with 1 U parathyroid extract/kg·h for 8 h. Plasma calcium rose 1 mg% and remained there for some time after the infusion was stopped. In five dogs, we removed the thyroid and parathyroid glands at the end of the infusion, and noted a rapid increase in plasma calcium (2 mg%) within 1 h. It was clear that removal of the glands had impaired control of hypercalcemia, but I failed to appreciate the importance of these observations. The point was also missed by Sanderson et al. (3) in 1960, when they observed impaired control of hypercalcemia in thyroparathyroidectomized dogs.

The significance became apparent in 1961, when we were studying the control of PTH secretion by perfusing the isolated thyroid/parathyroid glands of dogs with blood high or low in calcium. At that time it was felt that hypocalcemia was controlled by stimulation of PTH secretion, while hypercalcemia was controlled by suppressing it. In the critical experiment, shown in Fig. 1, we perfused these glands with high and low calcium blood and observed that the fall in plasma calcium during high calcium perfusion was very rapid, much more so than after parathyroidectomy. I finally removed the glands, expecting the level to fall, as predicted by current theory. To my surprise, it went up. It was at last clear that the high calcium perfusion had released a hypocalcemic hormone, which we called calcitonin because of its obvious role in controlling the level or "tone" of calcium in the blood (4). For various reasons, I thought that the hormone

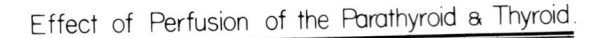

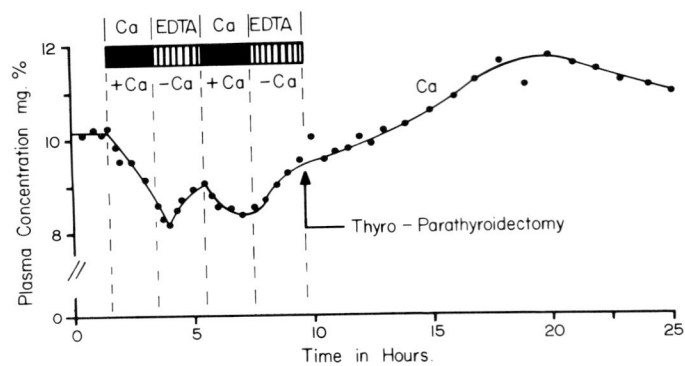

FIG. 1. Evidence which led to the recognition of calcitonin. Perfusion of the thyroid/parathyroid glands of the dog with high and low calcium blood. (From Copp et al., Endocrinology 70: 638–649, 1962.)

came from the parathyroids.

However, although the parathyroids of the dog do contain C cells and calcitonin, the principle source, as in other mammals, is the thyroid. Our results were confirmed by Kumar et al. (5) in 1963, and that same year Hirsch et al. (6) extracted the hormone from thyroid glands. They called it Thyrocalcitonin to indicate its gland of origin. Pearse (7) showed that calcitonin was produced by the C cells of the thyroid, which were derived from the ultimobranchial body of the embryo (8) and ultimately from the neural crest. With this information, we found calcitonin in the ultimobranchial glands of dogfish and chickens (9), whereas the thyroid had none. Meanwhile, the amino acid sequence for porcine (10) and human (11) calcitonin had been reported.

In the summer of 1968, we collected the ultimobranchials from half a million salmon. In a collaborative effort, the Armour Pharmaceutical Company processed them, we isolated pure salmon calcitonin. Niall et al. (12) determined the amino acid sequence, and the Sandoz Company in Basel synthesized it. Salmon calcitonin proved to be far more potent than porcine or human calcitonin, and is the form most widely used in human therapy.

The primary action of calcitonin is to lower plasma calcium by inhibiting bone resorption (13). While there is no indication that calcitonin is essential for life, it may have a role in protecting the skeleton in times of calcium stress, such as pregnancy and lactation. Clinically, it is used to treat hypercalcemia, Paget's disease, and osteoporosis.

Received May 7, 1992.

"Remembrance" articles discuss people and events as remembered by the author. The opinion(s) expressed are solely those of the writer and do not reflect the view of the Journal or The Endocrine Society.

Calcitonin is also a powerful pain suppressant, stimulating the secretion of the natural opiate, β-endorphin, and reducing the evoked potentials in important central pain pathways.

Because it inhibits bone resorption and relieves pain, calcitonin is now widely used in the treatment of bone disease, with world sales approaching one billion US dollars/annum, ranking it second only to insulin.

D. Harold Copp
Department of Physiology
University of British Columbia
Vancouver, British Columbia, Canada

References

1. **Fales FW** 1953 A micromethod for the determination of serum calcium. J Biol Chem 204:577–585
2. **Copp DH** 1967 Hormonal control of hypercalcemia. Historic development of the calcitonin concept. Am J Med 43:648–655
3. **Sanderson PH, Marshall F, Wilson R** 1960 Calcium and phosphorus homeostasis in the parathyroidectomized dog. Evaluation by means of EDTA and calcium tolerance tests. J Clin Invest 39:662–670
4. **Copp DH, Cameron EC, Cheney B, Davidson AGF, Henze K** 1962 Evidence for calcitonin—a new hormone from the parathyroid that lowers blood calcium. Endocrinology 70:638–649
5. **Kumar MA, Foster GV, MacIntyre I** 1963 Further evidence for calcitonin—a rapid acting hormone which lowers plasma calcium. Lancet 2:480–492
6. **Hirsch PF, Gauthier GF, Munson PL** 1963 Thyroid hypocalcemic principle and recurrent laryngeal nerve injury as factors affecting the response to parathyroidectomy in rats. Endocrinology 73:244–252
7. **Pearse AGE** 1966 The cytochemistry of the thyroid C cells and their relationship to calcitonin. Proc Roy Soc London (Biol) 170:71–80
8. **Pearse AGE, Cavalheira AF** 1967 Cytochemical evidence for an ultimobranchial origin of rodent thyroid C cells. Nature 214:929–923
9. **Copp DH, Cockcroft DW, Kueh Y** 1967 Calcitonin from ultimobranchial glands from dogfish and chickens. Science 158:924–926
10. **Potts JT, Niall HD, Keutmann HT, Brewer HB, Deftos LJ** 1968 The amino acid sequence of porcine thyrocalcitonin. Proc Natl Acad Sci USA 59:1321–1328
11. **Neher R, Riniker B, Rittel W, Zukor H** 1968 Mensehliches calcitonin III. Struktur von calcitonin M und D. Helv Chim Acta 51:1900–1905
12. **Niall HD, Keutmann HT, Copp DH, Potts JT** 1969 Amino acid sequence of salmon ultimobranchial calcitonin. Proc Natl Acad Sci USA 63:771–778
13. **Reynolds JJ** 1968 Inhibition by calcitonin of bone resorption induced *in vitro* by vitamin A. Proc Roy Soc London (Biol) 170:61–69

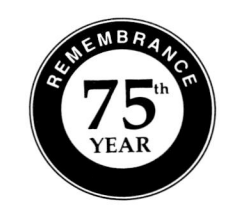

Remembrance: Gregory Pincus—Catalyst for Early Receptor Studies

Gregory Goodwin Pincus, President of The Endocrine Society in 1951–1952, was known as the progenitor of many things: the oral contraceptive, the Worcester Foundation for Experimental Biology, and the Laurentian Hormone Conference. Less widely appreciated was his salutary role in promoting acceptance of the concept of receptor-mediated steroid hormone action. His efforts, and a fortuitous combination of technical developments, were important progestational factors during the embryonic stages of receptor research.

In the mid 1950s, Herbert Jacobson and I, organic chemists in the Ben May Laboratory at the University of Chicago, were fascinated by the remarkable growth of the immature rat uterus after administration of nanogram amounts of an estrogenic hormone. At that time, two hypotheses had been proposed for the biochemical basis of this uterotrophic response. One postulated that the estrogen, being a flat molecule, could intercalate between base pairs in the nucleic acid structure and in some way alter template function or other activity of DNA. The other was the ingenious suggestion that the 17-hydroxyl group of estradiol, which, with placental enzymes undergoes reversible oxidation with either NAD or NADP, might serve as a hydrogen shuttle between these coenzymes to increase the levels of NADPH, a substance required in many biosynthetic reactions. This was the great era of enzymology. Most of the biochemical pathways of steroid metabolism had been elucidated, so an enzymatic "transhydrogenation" mechanism for estrogen action had strong appeal to biochemists and was widely accepted.

It seemed to us that consideration of an action mechanism required knowledge as to what happens to the steroid itself as it exerts its hormonal effect in target cells. Because estrogens are active in such small doses, it was apparent that, to obtain meaningful information concerning the fate of physiological amounts of administered steroid, one would need labeled hormone with a level of radioactivity far exceeding that of the ^{14}C-steroids available at the time. So with a graduate student, Gopi Gupta, and a postdoctoral fellow, Liselotte Closs, we set out in 1956 to prepare 6,7-^{3}H-estradiol of high specific activity from the catalytic reduction of 6-dehydroestradiol with carrier-free tritium.

To be sure that all the steroid molecules were labeled, it was necessary to use a microhydrogenator that could measure the uptake of tritium by the double bond but keep the total gas volume to a minimum. But the smallest apparatus we could devise still required 50 Ci tritium gas, more than

Received February 26, 1992.
"Remembrance" articles discuss people and events as remembered by the author. The opinion(s) expressed are solely those of the writer and do not reflect the view of the Journal or The Endocrine Society.

was permitted on our campus. Fortunately, at the Argonne National Laboratory 15 miles away, Kenneth Wilzbach and Louis Kaplan had the required high level facilities, which they generously made available for our hydrogenation experiments. So we synthesized our "hot" estradiol, and learned how to purify and store it with minimal decomposition.

To measure the ^{3}H-steroid in tissue specimens, we needed a simple technique to convert the tritium to a form that could be conveniently counted. Here, again, we were aided by fortuitous events. Weldon Brown, in our Chemistry Department, had developed a procedure for converting tritium in organic compounds to tritiated water by combustion with cupric oxide, and we found this to work well with dried tissues. At the urging of Leon Jacobson of the Department of Medicine, Lyle Packard in our electronics shop had devised an automated apparatus to measure carbon-14 and tritium by liquid scintillation counting, and he had just formed a company to build these instruments. We were fortunate to obtain the eighth Tricarb counter produced, which enabled us to carry out experiments with large numbers of replicate specimens so as to determine reliably the fate of ^{3}H-estradiol in tissues of the immature rat.

After devoting a year to the preparation of labeled hormone and the development of analytical procedures, we were ready to begin our studies. By late 1957 it was clear that "target" tissues, such as uterus, vagina, and anterior pituitary, contained hitherto unrecognized components that took up and retained estradiol against a marked concentration gradient with the blood. We decided to present what to us were exciting findings at the 4th International Congress of Biochemistry in Vienna in August 1958. This report met with little interest. Five people were in the audience, three of whom were other speakers. It seemed that our session coincided with a major symposium on hormone action, where a thousand scientists came to hear about the participation of steroid hormones in enzymatic reactions.

Somehow Gregory Pincus learned of our experiments and invited us to describe them at a conference on steroids and cancer that he was organizing in Vermont for the autumn of 1959. By then we had more data which generated greater interest, and in the same year there was also a report by Glascock and Hoekstra in England of similar concentration of the synthetic estrogen, hexestrol, by reproductive tissues of goats and sheep. But there still were many who doubted that these results had anything to do with hormone action, for it was difficult to see their relation to enzymology. In fact, one eminent biochemist told me that he could have little interest in binding studies unless we identified some kind of enzymatic activity for the binding substance.

Gregory Pincus was not dismayed by such reservations,

and he invited us to report our findings to a wider audience at the 1961 Laurentian Hormone Conference. By then our group had added two postdoctoral fellows, James Flesher and Narendra Saha, and we demonstrated that estradiol is taken up by the immature rat uterus without apparent chemical change. To rule out the possibility of reversible oxidation-reduction at the 17-position with equilibrium favoring the reduced state, we synthesized 17α-^{3}H-estradiol and showed that, after rats were given a mixture of the 6,7- and 17-^{3}H-hormones, the estradiol in the uterus had the same ratio of the two components as that administered. Thus, it was clear that estradiol does not undergo oxidation-reduction or other metabolic transformation as it stimulates growth of the immature rat uterus.

After the Laurentian Conference, the importance of steroid binding in hormone action was rapidly accepted, although there still was some reluctance, especially on the part of editors, to refer to the binding entities as receptors. We had also reported at the 1961 meeting that a known estrogen antagonist, MER-25, unlike antiuterotrophic agents related to progesterone, prevented the uptake of estradiol. We then used varying doses of a similar antagonist, nafoxidine, to demonstrate a close correlation between reduction in steroid binding and inhibition of uterine growth. These findings, along with our observation that blockage of the uterine growth response with puromycin or actinomycin-D did not prevent hormone binding, gave evidence that the binding substances actually are receptors, and that their interaction with the steroid is an early and necessary step in hormone action.

In 1965, Gregory Pincus asked our group, which now included Eugene DeSombre and Peter Jungblut, to present a summary of all our studies at an international conference in Tokyo under the title: "Estrogen receptors in target tissues" (1). This was the first time that we were able to include the word "receptor" in our title. Even so, a friendly polemic about the use of this term still existed in 1968 (2), whereas as late as 1973, at a breast cancer meeting in Brussels, an eminent elderly pharmacologist shook his finger under my nose and shouted: "How dare you speak of receptors when they aren't even in a membrane?"

After the introduction by Toft and Gorski in 1966 of ultracentrifugation techniques for characterizing estradiol-receptor complexes, we were able in 1968 to distinguish two forms of the steroid-binding component and to show in 1971 that an important role of the steroid is to convert the native receptor protein to an activated state that can associate with target cell nuclei to enhance RNA synthesis. With the identification by many workers of intracellular binding proteins for other classes of steroid hormones and the demonstration that steroid-induced transformation to an active modulator of transcription is a general property of all these substances, little doubt remained that these binding proteins mediate steroid hormone action and qualify as true receptors.

Gregory Pincus died in 1967, just as hormone-receptor interactions were beginning to be identified for all classes of steroids. No doubt he would have enjoyed this verification of the importance of hormone binding, and he certainly would have been thrilled by the spectacular recent success of molecular biologists in elucidating receptor structure and the precise molecular details of the earlier phenomenology. For those of us who were involved in those primitive stages, the interest and support by Gregory Pincus for a concept alien to the thinking at that time will always be a fond remembrance.

Elwood V. Jensen
Institute for Hormone and Fertility Research
University of Hamburg, Germany

References

1. **Jensen EV, Jacobson HI, Flesher JW, Saha NN, Gupta GN, Smith S, Colucci V, Shiplacoff D, Neumann HG, DeSombre ER, Jungblut PW** 1966 Estrogen receptors in target tissues. In: Pincus G, Nakao T, Tait JF (eds) Steroid Dynamics. Academic Press, New York, pp 133–156
2. **Wurtman RJ** 1968 Estrogen receptor: ambiguities in the use of this term. Science 159:1261; Jensen EV ibid.

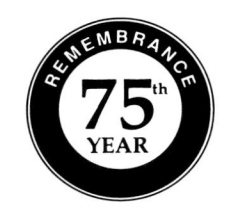

Remembrance: The Introduction of Molecular Biology and Receptors into the Study of Hormone Action

The roots of molecular biology date back to the early 1950s when studies of nucleic acid chemistry led to the first structural models of DNA, and genetic studies of bacteria led to our first models of regulation of gene expression. Endocrinology, at that time, was fixated on the previous decade's discoveries of the metabolic enzymes and the role of cofactors in regulating intermediary metabolism. In particular, steroid hormones were studied as metabolic substrates that were expected to have critical metabolites, which in turn were likely to be cofactors in an essential metabolic pathway. The culmination of this line of reasoning came in the form of the steroid-dependent transhydrogenase theory of the late 1950s. This theory proposed that hormonal steroids acted as oxidation-reduction cofactors in the transfer of reducing equivalents from NADH to NADP. Whereas there were some reservations expressed about the transhydrogenase theory, it was generally accepted as explaining the biological response to estrogens and other steroids.

Two new lines of steroid hormone research, represented by a small minority of investigators, also were underway in the 1950s. The research of these investigators was to lead to the demise of the transhydrogenase theory and to the development of current models of steroid hormone action. Studies of tissue and cell uptake of steroid hormones had been hindered by the low specific activity of the radioactive C14 steroids; all that were available at the time. This in turn necessitated the use of large, nonphysiological doses of the steroid in either animals or tissue incubations. The introduction of tritium-labeled steroids had a major impact on steroid hormone research. Preparing and counting tritiated compounds in the 1950s was no trivial matter. This predated commercial sources of tritiated compounds, and scintillation counters were just in the development stages. Elwood Jensen was a young organic chemist in the Ben May Laboratories at the University of Chicago who incorporated the available techniques of tritiating and counting estrogenic steroids, which made these early studies of hormone action possible. Jensen's studies, in conjunction with H. Jacobson and others, were undertaken when receptors were only a theoretical concept that pharmacologists talked about but for which there were no experimental observations (1). No one had actually studied directly a receptor of any kind up to that time. For example, the research model for neurotransmitter receptors in the 1950s and the 1960s was the enzyme acetylcholine esterase. As mentioned above, the steroids were also thought to function by interacting with other enzymes.

Into this scientific scene came the first of Jensen's reports, a paper presented at the 1958 International Biochemistry meetings in Vienna. Jensen's paper was delivered in a session of short reports. It is ironic that Jensen's paper was scheduled concurrently with a major symposium on steroid hormones and transhydrogenases. Obviously, everyone who worked on steroid hormones was at the symposium except for a small band (five) of Elwood's friends who showed up for his presentation. Those five listeners heard the report that presaged the demise of the transhydrogenase theory and introduced a new era in the study of steroid hormone action. These early studies of steroid hormone receptors laid the ground rules for all the hormone receptor studies that were to follow; thus Elwood Jensen and his colleagues were the creators of the modern concept of receptors.

Another major thread of investigation beginning in the 1950s was the development of molecular biology. The Watson-Crick structure of DNA and, perhaps more importantly, the Jacob, Monod, and Pardee studies of regulation of gene expression in prokaryotes led to an early interest by a number of investigators in the regulation of gene expression in eukaryotes. Gerald Mueller of the McArdle Laboratories at the University of Wisconsin-Madison was one whose interest was aroused, and he immediately began to investigate certain aspects of nucleic acid and protein synthesis in uterine tissue of the estrogen-stimulated rat (2). He and his associates were able to demonstrate that estrogen markedly increased overall RNA synthesis within hours after estrogen treatment. They also found that protein synthesis increased early, suggesting that the entire gene expression system might be stimulated by estrogens. This led to the model of steroid hormone action presented by Mueller at the 1957 Laurentian Hormone Conference and reprinted here as Fig. 1. Mueller used the terminology of prokaryote gene expression; inducers, antiinducers, unmasking, *etc.*, but it is clear that he had a vision that steroid hormones, by interacting with specific chromatin proteins, played a critical role in the process of gene regulation.

A recurring problem with these early studies was the inability to work with specific proteins or gene products because of the lack of suitable methods. I can remember, as a postdoctoral fellow in Mueller's laboratory, the morning when Gerry came into the laboratory highly excited by a paper he had read the evening before. The paper reported that a new antibiotic, Puromycin, was effective in blocking protein synthesis in animal cells. Mueller saw the potential of this inhibitor and used the antibiotic to block protein synthesis and all the known responses to estrogen in uterine tissue (3). He thus demonstrated that specific responses to estrogen depended on prior protein synthesis. This impli-

---

Received April 1, 1992.

"Remembrance" articles discuss people and events as remembered by the author. The opinion(s) expressed are solely those of the writer and do not reflect the view of the Journal or The Endocrine Society.

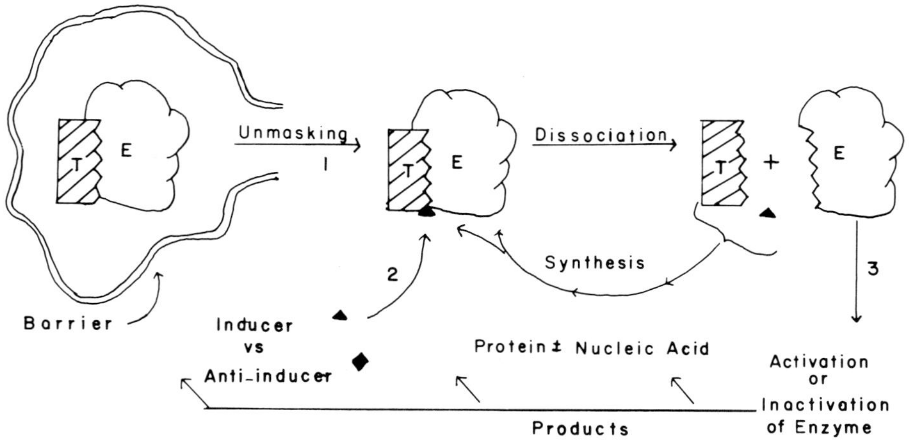

FIG. 1. A scheme depicting possible sites of hormonal regulation of induced biosynthesis. T, Template; E, enzyme; 1, 2, or 3, possible sites of hormone action. (Reprinted with permission of the authors; Ref. 2.).

cated estrogen as inducing the synthesis of specific proteins just as inducers did in bacterial cells, and led to later studies that showed estrogen induction of specific gene expression.

In the 30 plus years since these investigations by Jensen's and Mueller's laboratories, their original ideas have been confirmed and extended in great measure. The extent of the receptor gene superfamily certainly has been a surprise and the complexity of gene expression regulation in animal cells was not predicted. However, these two pioneers made observations and predictions that served as major turning points for subsequent research into hormone action. Their influence also illustrates that science is not a democratic institution in which a majority vote is conclusive but rather is a continuing process in which minority positions can eventually prevail.

Jack Gorski
Department of Biochemistry and Animal Sciences
University of Wisconsin
Madison, Wisconsin

References

1. **Jensen EV, Jacobson HI** 1960 Fate of steroid estrogens in target tissues. In: Pincus G, Vollner E (eds) Biological Activities of Steroids in Relation to Cancer. Academic Press, New York, pp 161–178
2. **Mueller GC, Herranen AM, Jervell KF** 1957 Studies on the mechanism of action of estrogens. Recent Prog Hormone Res 4:95–139
3. **Mueller GC, Gorski J, Aizawa Y** 1961 The role of protein synthesis in early estrogen action. Proc Natl Acad Sci USA 47:164–169

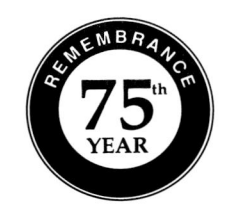

Remembrance: The Story of Inhibin—The Melbourne Version

Because a group of us working in Melbourne, Australia, were fortunate enough to contribute significantly to research on inhibin and its related peptides, it seemed appropriate, as part of the Remembrance project to set down a few key events in the history culminating in the first successful purification of inhibin from bovine follicular fluid, by Robertson et al. (1).

de Kretser et al. (2) provided important beginnings as a result of their work on testicular structure and function, prepared for his thesis for Melbourne University's Degree of Doctor of Medicine in the late 1960s. In collaborative studies involving Bryan Hudson (2) whose influence throughout was crucial, Pincus Taft and myself, and applying the recently developed FSH RIA, we showed that some men with severe seminiferous tubule failure had selective elevations in circulating FSH and postulated that there was indeed a seminiferous tubule factor which was deficient in such individuals and which corresponded to inhibin as originally postulated by McCullagh 40 yr earlier (3).

In 1972 I began a sabbatical year in the laboratory of Dr. Paul Franchimont, in Liege, Belgium. Paul's group had been pioneers in the development of FSH RIAs and reported similar findings in seminiferous tubule failure (4). Paul had made a very important observation in addition, that the injection of normal seminal plasma into castrate male rats could induce selective lowering of their elevated FSH levels, that seminal plasma from men with oligospermia was less effective, and that seminal plasma from men with azoospermia lacked the inhibitory activity (5). This was an important stimulus to the continued search for inhibin, which both the Melbourne and Liege groups pursued subsequently. Two other key people with early involvement in the research on inhibin were Victor Lee and Ted Keogh (6). They infused bovine testicular extracts into castrate sheep and obtained critical evidence that FSH but not LH was suppressed, while similarly prepared liver extracts were ineffective. George Rennie (6) provided the statistical expertise in the analysis of the data.

Eddie et al. (7) developed a dispersed cultured pituitary cell bioassay system, in which inhibin containing biological extracts suppressed LHRH stimulated FSH and LH release. The assay was applied to efforts at purifying the biological activity, from testicular extracts and rete testis fluid, in which Gordon Baker was involved, but this proved quite elusive. Biological activity was continually lost from various chromatographic systems. At this point Hugh Niall and Geoff Tregear joined the Howard Florey Institute (where Hudson, Keogh, Baker, Eddie were working) while deKretser and I worked at Prince Henry's Hospital Medical Research Centre. There I had been joined by Russell Scott (8), a New Zealand Ph.D student, who modified the pituitary cell bioassay so as to measure the cellular content of FSH and LH, rather than their release, thus allowing the assay of FSH containing fluids and contributing significantly to the elimination of nonspecific effects in the assay. This system proved robust and capable of handling multiple samples and was used for the collaborative attempts to purify inhibin, involving Niall, Tregear and Hudson at the Florey and deKretser and myself at Monash University and at Prince Henry's.

In late 1978, an amicable agreement was reached that each Group would proceed largely independently with efforts to purify inhibin. We would continue to share inhibin standards, but while the Florey team would persist with rete testis fluid we would switch to bovine ovarian follicular fluid, readily obtained from the abbatoir. David Robertson had now joined us from an extensive apprenticeship with Egon Dicsfalusy at the Karolinska and brought a new degree of rigor to the purification process. It was to his outstanding efforts that we can attribute the ultimate success of purifying first 58 kilodalton and then 31 kilodalton bovine inhibin. Of great importance to that success was the involvement of two other collaborators, then working at St. Vincent's Hospital School of Medical Research, Frank Morgan and Milton Hearn. Frank provided us with expertise in the techniques of preparative polyacrylamide gel electrophoresis, and Milton in reversed-phase HPLC, both of which were essential steps in achieving the purification. They, together with Dick Wettenhall, provided the protein sequencing techniques to allow the initiation of the cloning of the hormone, for which we sought the assistance of a commercial partner, Biotechnology Australia, from which Rob Forage in particular provided invaluable input. Dobos et al. (9) had in fact made the first attempts to use HPLC for the purification. Lynda Foulds and Lorraine Leversha provided high quality technical expertise in the whole purification procedure.

A fundamental element in the entire endeavour was the long standing tradition of collaboration across scientific institutions in Melbourne and it was the strength of that collaboration which led to the ultimately successful outcome. Our group devoted essentially all of our resources to the problem and were supported by significant grants from the World Health Organisation Special Programme in Human Reproduction, the Ford Foundation, and the Australian National Health and Medical Research Council. Participants in Melbourne provided a unique combination of expertise in fundamental techniques of protein chemistry, animal physi-

---

Received February 21, 1992.

"Remembrance" articles discuss people and events as remembered by the author. The opinion(s) expressed are solely those of the writer and do not reflect the view of the Journal or The Endocrine Society.

ology (in which Jock Findlay contributed substantially), and human clinical investigation. David de Kretser and I ran regular meetings of which careful minutes were kept, charting the progress of what was often a highly frustrating and difficult project. We were single minded about the need to maintain a long range strategic plan to achieve the purification of inhibin.

It is sobering for me to reflect on the ultimate reason for my involvement in all this, I had sailed to the United States aboard the Queen Mary in January 1963 from the United Kingdom originally intending to join the late Fred Bartter for further training in steroid hormone physiology. Just before departure, Bryan Hudson had advised me to switch into protein hormone research and to learn RIA, which he saw as the new direction. I applied to work with Peter Condliffe where I began to learn from him and Harold Edelhoch about proteins and sat at the feet of the master, Jesse Roth, fresh from Sol Berson and Ros Yalow's lab, to learn the art of RIA, which led me to the gonadotropins and inhibin.

Henry Burger
Prince Henry's Institute of Medical Research
Monash Medical Centre
Clayton, Victoria

References

1. **Robertson DM, Foulds LM, Leversha L, Morgan FJ, Hearn MTW, Burger HG, Wettenhall REH, de Kretser DM** 1985 Isolation of inhibin from bovine follicular fluid. Biochem Biophys Res Commun 126:220–226
2. **de Kretser DM, Burger HG, Fortune D, Hudson B, Long AR, Paulsen CA, Taft HP** 1972 Hormonal, histological and chromosomal studies in adult males with testicular disorders. J Clin Endocrinol Metab 35:392–401
3. **McCullagh DR** 1932 Dual control of testis. Science 76:19–20
4. **Franchimont P, Millet D, Vendrely E, Letawe J, Legros JJ, Netter A** 1972 Relationship between spermatogenesis and serum gonadotropin levels in azoospermia and oligospermia. J Clin Endocrinol Metab 34:1003–1008
5. **Scott RS, Burger HG** 1981 An inverse relationship exists between seminal plasma inhibin and serum FSH in man. J Clin Endocrinol Metab 52:796–803
6. **Keogh EJ, Lee VWK, Rennie GC, Burger HG, Hudson B, de Kretser DM** 1976 Selective suppression of FSH by testicular extracts. Endocrinology 98:997–1004
7. **Eddie LW, Baker HWG, Higginson RE, Hudson B** 1979 A Bioassay for inhibin using pituitary cell cultures. J Endocrinol 81:49–60
8. **Scott RS, Burger HG, Quigg H** 1980 A simple and rapid *in vitro* bioassay for inhibin. Endocrinology 107:1536–1542
9. **Dobos M, Burger HG, Hearn MTW, Morgan FJ** 1983 Isolation of ovine follicular fluid inhibin using reversed-phase liquid chromatography. Mol Cell Endocrinol 31:187–198

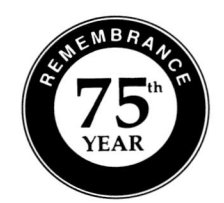

Remembrance: Excerpta Memorabilia

1932–1933. Hypophysectomy—Greep

Only because I had to stay up most of the night at the lab in Madison (tending to my adrenalectomized rats with my own adrenal cortical extract) did I become aware that Roy, with Eunice's help, was trying to remove the pituitary from rats. Only P. E. Smith of Columbia was performing it successfully. Roy Hertz, after his B.S. in zoology at Madison, had gone to Columbia for his Master's, but was unable to get to see Smith do the operation. Now Hertz was back at Madison for his doctorate and was working as Hisaw's research assistant.

After many such nights, when Roy and Eunice knew why I was there, and I learned what they were doing, Eunice pledged me to secrecy. Roy did not want "the Boss" or others to learn that he was trying but might fail. However, he succeeded, with 30-day-old rats, parapharyngeal approach, a hand drill which a friend had made, and an oral suction tube (with a side "catch"). I have often wondered how many rat "pits" Ray may have swallowed!

From then on Roy was Hisaw's "boy."

1935. Hisaw's offer from Harvard

As we walked down Euclid Avenue to afternoon Anatomy meetings at Washington University, Hisaw found a telegram with the mail he had picked up at the hotel after lunch. He stopped and read it aloud, an offer to come to Harvard at $12,000 per year plus (I forget—at so much per semester for lectures to Radcliffe students). This would virtually double his Wisconsin salary, which, I had accidentally learned earlier during a post-doc summer research at Madison, was $7700. I can't recall whether I said it or just thought it: "Dr. Hisaw, I hope you stay at Wisconsin!"

But at Harvard he also developed an outstanding group of doctorate students: Roy Talmadge, Mike Zarrow, Bill Money, Hilton Salhanick, Ted Astwood, *et al*. Yet at Wisconsin his research had yielded Relaxin, FSH, LH, and hard-working students: R. K. Rolly Meyer, Kip Weichert, Roy Greep, Sam Leonard, Art Hellbaum, Roy Hertz, Bob Kroc, and others.

1941. Kinsey—The Journal of Clinical Endocrinology (1)

Yes! Kinsey's first publication in the field of human sexual behavior was in one of our journals! How come? I was teaching endocrinology at Indiana University in the Zoology Department. Alfred Kinsey had recruited me to come to IU to take over his biology course (after my doctorate with Hisaw) so that he (Kinsey) could have more time for his field trips to collect galls off oak trees for their entrapped wasp larvae.

Some years later, however, the Women Students' Organization petitioned President Wells to organize a course in Marriage and The Family. Our bachelor president said he would have to appoint a faculty committee to determine how this should be done and who would be involved. He asked for suggestions from the women students, and Kinsey was among those suggested. "But," said Wells, "why Kinsey—he studies gall wasps!" Their answer was that as a biology teacher he had a reputation of giving straight, frank, and useful answers if personal questions were asked.

By 1940 Kinsey had essentially stopped his gall wasp research and had been chairman of the faculty group giving the Marriage course for students over the age of 21 or with parental consent!!! I (R.L.K.) was one of the lecturers in the course.

Students could request private interviews with any of the dozen or so lecturers; this resulted in Kinsey's collection of case histories.

When a paper by Glass *et al.* appeared in 1940 (2) I drew it to Kinsey's attention. I was doubtful about their conclusion of hormonal differences between homo- and heterosexual males. Numbers were small, samples were pooled, and their statistics seemed poor (2). Frank Edmondson, Prof. of Astronomy (an expert statistician) agreed. I was also aware that Kinsey's case histories of males would be in disagreement with the authors' conclusions.

So, Kinsey's reply was accepted by the editors of the new journal in volume 1 of *The Journal of Clinical Endocrinology* (1).

This recalls research of Carroll Pfeiffer, Yale Ph.D., Prof. at the medical school in Puerto Rico, who published in the 1930s and 1940s on experimental hormonal effects in pregnant rats, resulting in altered sexual behavior of their offspring.

And now we have the reports of Simon LeVay on hypothalamic differences between hetero- and homosexual men!

Thus, while there may be no hormonal differences between sexual orientations in men, there may be biological-neurological differences! Kinsey would enjoy the distinction!!!!

Robert L. Kroc
Santa Barbara, California

Received June 2, 1992.

"Remembrance" articles discuss people and events as remembered by the author. The opinion(s) expressed are solely those of the writer and do not reflect the view of the Journal or The Endocrine Society.

References

1. **Kinsey AC** 1941 Criteria for a hormonal explanation of the homosexual. J Clin Endocrinol 1:424–428
2. **Glass SJ, Deuel HJ, Wright CA** 1940 Sex hormone studies in male homosexuality. Endocrinology 26:590–594

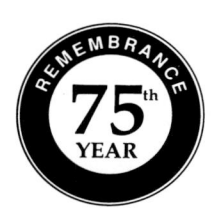

The Development of the Role of Hormones in Development—a Double Remembrance

Comparative endocrinology: the thyroid-PRL relationship in amphibian development

Comparative endocrinology virtually originated with the emergence of experimental endocrinology. The second decade of this century witnessed seminal contributions by Friedrich Gudernatsch, Bennett M. Allen and Philip E. Smith, all of whom used the amphibian (frog) tadpole as their experimental animal. Their challenge was to discover what was responsible for the dramatic events connoted by the term metamorphosis, wherein an aquatic larva (tadpole) generally becomes a semiterrestrial adult: gills and tails are resorbed, legs differentiate, oral and intestinal structures change. These pioneers extirpated and transplanted various glandular structures, ultimately elucidating the pituitary-thyroid axis and assigning to the thyroid hormone the central role of inducing both progressive and regressive developmental changes.

Critical to this elucidation was microsurgical expertise. B. M. Allen's particular expertise involved the use of "needle knives," wherein the head of a needle was broken off and the broken edge of the shaft was honed to a beveled angular knife—sharp and pointed. I learned this high technology before World War II at the University of California at Los Angeles, as a National Youth Administration-supported undergraduate assistant to Professor Allen, a gruff and dignified gentleman who appreciated my ability but not my depressed economic status. From time to time, he would take me to a fancy Westwood Village restaurant (near UCLA) for lunch and suggest a nice green salad, when what I needed most was substance and not cellulose. Despite my weakened condition, I used his technique to hypophysectomize hundreds of local salamanders. With graduation, I deserted his aegis and his research area for redder fields (mammalian reproductive endocrinology) but never deserted my feelings of respect and affection for my first patron.

The sigh of relief with which I had left amphibian glands behind me lasted some 25 yr or so when my interests in PRL and the evolution of its functions, perked by the arrival of Charles S. Nicoll as a postdoctoral fellow, and sustained by collaboration with him and my colleagues Richard C. Strohman and Paul Licht, led me back to the amphibian and the discovery, simultaneously with William S. Etkin, that the control of amphibian metamorphosis was not unihormonal, with thyroid hormone favoring metamorphosis and the emergence of adult characteristics, but bihormonal, with PRL opposing metamorphosis and favoring larval growth and retention of larval characteristics (1). Both Etkin and I were struck by the analogy with the well established bihormonal control of insect metamorphosis by ecdysone and juvenile hormone. The thyroid hormone-PRL antagonism later proved to have implications for phenomena distantly removed from tadpole development such as mammary gland development (which Dharm V. Singh and I in Berkeley and Indraneel Mittra in London independently investigated in the mouse). Studies on salamanders, some of which have a second metamorphosis (George Wald's term) back to aquatic life (PRL-induced "water drive"), further substantiated the antagonistic thyroid hormone-PRL relation (2). To update the situation fully, the control over amphibian metamorphosis is best described as multihormonal, as the role of other hormones, especially corticosteroids, has been recognized (by Sakae Kikuyama and Charles S. Nicoll; 3, 4).

If there is a lesson to be learned from this remembrance, it is that biological explanation is never complete. Even as obvious a phenomenon as the thyroid control of metamorphosis, schoolchild in its simplicity and long accepted as textbook dogma, has become complicated by the recognition of hormonal interactions and the discovery of new roles for old hormones. In no manner could the growth/differentiation activity of PRL have been subsumed by an understanding of its mammotropic/lactogenic activity (although the converse may have some elements of credibility).

Mammalian endocrinology: the developmental effects of estrogens

In the 1950s, Professor Kiyoshi Takewaki, distinguished member of the Japan Academy and pioneering experimental endocrinologist in his country, brought the concept of "persistent estrus" in rats to the attention of endocrinologists. Arriving at Berkeley as a young postdoctoral in 1960, his former student Noboru Takasugi (now President of Yokohama City University) sought to establish the existence of this phenomenon in mice. Although persistent vaginal cornification and stratification characterize the affected mice, persistent estrus is in fact a misnomer: the mice do not show estrous behavior and they are anovulatory. One of Takewaki's findings was that the persistent changes in rats were abolished by ovariectomy. When Takasugi ovariectomized those mice receiving higher doses of estradiol neonatally, the vaginal changes persisted, much to his consternation (5). Further endocrinectomies (adrenalectomy, hypophysectomy) failed to eliminate these changes. It became apparent that estrogen had acted at the level of the target organ, possibly selecting a cell population (heterotopic) which would ordinarily disappear in ontogenetic development (or selecting a

---

Received March 23, 1992.

"Remembrance" articles discuss people and events as remembered by the author. The opinion(s) expressed are solely those of the writer and do not reflect the view of the Journal or The Endocrine Society.

heterotopic mesenchyme which instructed the overlying epithelium to differentiate in an abnormal fashion). Thus, the effect of the estrogen was essentially teratogenic, and ultimately led to the appearance of dysplastic, preneoplastic, and neoplastic lesions. This permanent, ovary-independent effect represented a new phenomenon in regard to estrogen action.

Ten years later, Arthur Herbst described several cases of vaginal clear cell adenocarcinoma in young women, a rare variety of cancer which until then had been encountered in postmenopausal women, whose mothers had ingested diethylstilbestrol [(DES) a nonsteroidal synthetic estrogen] during the first trimester of pregnancy. This clinical DES syndrome was a human parallel to the murine syndrome, and the neonatal mouse thus provided a preexistent model for the human disorder (6-8).

There is a critical period for the action of estrogen which leads to vaginal neoplasia in both human and mouse: before the end of the first trimester in the human, before day 3 or 4 in the neonatal mouse. Genital tract maturation in human and mouse is roughly equivalent at these two times. (In the rat, it has since been shown that late prenatal exposure to estrogen will induce changes comparable to those induced in the neonatal mouse.) A second major aspect derived from the mouse studies is the recognition that the potency of the estrogen during development may have little relation to its potency in postnatal life established by *in vivo* and *in vitro* assays, including receptor assays. Weak estrogens such as plant estrogens may be strong stimuli during mouse development. Even so-called antiestrogens (generally also weak agonists), such as tamoxifen and clomiphene, induce pathological consequences similar to what is seen after neonatal exposure to natural estrogens, steroidal and nonsteroidal (plant estrogens), and synthetic estrogens such as DES (9).

Although the danger of fetal exposure to DES and other recognized estrogens is now minimal (and has been since the early '70s), the environment contains synthetic chemical agents, such as some dioxins and PCBs, which like derivatives of the now-banned DDT, may prove to be weakly estrogenic in standard assays. Extrapolating from what is known about the developmental effects of other weak estrogens, there should be concern about the DES-like role that these environmental estrogens could play if ingested (or inhaled) extensively by mothers during a critical period of development of their offspring *in utero*.

What is striking about the neonatal mouse is the promiscuity of the responsiveness of its developing genital tract. In addition to its sensitivity to estrogens, weak and strong, and antiestrogens, the differentiating female system responds in part similarly to androgens and to progestins. The nature of the estrogen receptor, indeed of the steroid receptor family, during organogenesis is largely unknown. Is the ontogenetically primitive estrogen receptor nondiscriminatory or are there "orphan" receptors present which act as transcription factors and lead to similar responses? This is an area as rich in its challenges to the molecular endocrinologist as it is rich in its implications for the reproductive biologist, the tumor biologist, and the environmental biologist.

This remembrance offers a striking example of serendipity in endocrinological research. An experiment conducted with the mundane intent of repeating in a second species what had been established in a first species led to the discovery of the profound developmental effect of estrogen, opening a story which, regrettably, threatens to continue for some time to come.

Howard A. Bern
Professor of Integrative Biology, Emeritus
  and member of the Group in Endocrinology
  the Cancer Research Laboratory and
  the Bodega Marine Laboratory
University of California, Berkeley

References

1. **Bern HA, Nicoll CS, Strohman RC** 1967 Prolactin and tadpole growth. Proc Soc Exp Biol Med 126:518–521
2. **Bern HA, Nicoll CS** 1968 The comparative endocrinology of prolactin. Recent Prog Horm Res 24:681–720
3. **Kikuyama S, Yamamoto K** 1988 Prolactin and amphibian metamorphosis. In: Hoshino K (ed) Prolactin Gene Family and its Receptors. Excerpta Medica, Amsterdam, pp 359–366
4. **White BA, Nicoll CS** 1981 Hormonal control of amphibian metamorphosis. In: Gilbert LI, Frieden E (eds) Metamorphosis: a Problem in Development. Plenum Press, New York, pp 363–396
5. **Takasugi N, Bern HA, DeOme KB** 1962 Persistent vaginal cornification in mice. Science 138:438–439
6. **Herbst AL, Bern HA** (eds) 1981 Developmental Effects of Diethylstilbestrol (DES) in Pregnancy. Thieme-Stratton, New York
7. **Mori T, Nagasawa H** (eds) 1988 Toxicity of Hormones in Perinatal Life. CRC Press, Boca Raton
8. **Bern HA**, Diethylstilbestrol (DES) syndrome: present status of animal and human studies. In: Li J, Nandi S, Li SA (eds) Hormonal Carcinogenesis. Springer-Verlag, New York, 1992, pp 1–8
9. **Bern HA**, The fragile fetus. In: Colborn T, Clement C (eds) Chemically Induced Alterations in Sexual and Functional Development: The Wildlife/Human Connection. Princeton Scientific Publishing, Princeton, 1992, pp 9–15

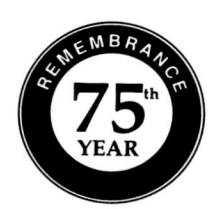

Remembrance: Growing Up with the Pineal Gland: Early Recollections

An understanding of the biochemistry and the physiology of the pineal gland entered the 1960s at the lower end of the proverbial scientific totem pole. In general, most endocrinologists considered the gland an evolutionary relic whose function had either run its course or had never even evolved. I recall listening to a seminar presentation by a fellow graduate student in 1961 during which he summarized what was, or more correctly what wasn't, known about an organ then usually referred to as the pineal body or epiphysis cerebri. I left the presentation convinced the pineal would not likely be a productive research area to enter and I clearly dismissed the entire idea until I was inadvertently drawn to it after I completed my doctoral education.

The decade of the 1960s had been, however, ushered in by a very important discovery by Aaron Lerner and colleagues (1, 2) at Yale who, after an expensive and tedious effort, had succeeded in isolating and characterizing melatonin. An exceedingly small quantity (less than 100 μg) of melatonin, now known to be the chief hormonal product of the pineal gland, was initially isolated from an estimated 250,000 bovine pineals. This group also hypothesized that it was a derivative of serotonin and, in fact, they named melatonin accordingly. Thus, the term melatonin is a combination of the terms serotonin (from which melatonin is derived) and melanin (on which melatonin acts to lighten the skin of amphibians, reptiles, and fishes). The alternate name for the newly discovered hormone was apparently yalin, after Lerner's home university; I'm glad he selected the name melatonin.

Other than that it contained melatonin, little was known of the pineal gland when Julie Axelrod and Herb Weissbach and their colleagues attacked the problem of determining the metabolic steps by which serotonin is transformed into melatonin. In 1960, Axelrod and Weissbach (3) surmised that the biosynthesis of melatonin proceeded via the acetylation of serotonin to N-acetylserotonin which was then O-methylated to melatonin. They soon succeeded in enzymatically converting N-acetylserotonin to melatonin with the melatonin-forming enzyme being designated hydroxyindole-O-methyltransferase (HIOMT) (4).

Besides these findings, the control of pineal serotonin metabolism and melatonin synthesis by the light-dark cycle (LD) proved to be an important finding. Bill Quay (5) in 1963 found that the quantity of serotonin within the pineal gland varied over a 24-h LD cycle with serotonin levels always being lower at night than during the day; essentially simultaneously, Dick Wurtman, working with Axelrod, demonstrated that the melatonin forming ability of the pineal gland, as indicated by the activity of HIOMT, was stimulated by darkness (6). Also entering on the scene at this time was Sol Snyder, who with Axelrod and Wurtman, worked out the details of the role of light and darkness in regulating pineal HIOMT activity and confirming the essential position of the sympathetic innervation to the organ in carrying information about the LD cycle to the gland (7). The important upshot of these biochemical studies was that melatonin production by the pineal gland was believed to be stimulated by darkness and suppressed during the light.

At the time the biochemical details were being clarified at NIH, Roger Hoffman and myself (at Edgewood Arsenal, MD), were working with the Syrian hamster in experiments related to the physiology of the pineal gland. This proved a fortuitous choice since this species happens to be extremely photoperiodic. Interestingly, I had arrived at Edgewood Arsenal (to fulfill a military obligation as a Reserve Officer's Training Corps officer) in March of 1964, fresh from receiving my doctoral degree, and I was charged by the commanding office of the medical laboratories to investigate "the physiological consequences of photoperiodic and temperature manipulations." By October of the same year, Hoffman and I had found that the reproductive system of the hamster is readily inhibited when they are kept under short day conditions and, more importantly, that the suppressive effect of darkness is prevented if the pineal gland had been surgically removed from the animals. I recall well the day as being Friday, and the immediate excitement that filled the laboratory when the gonads of the intact and pinealectomized hamsters were compared. The differences were so dramatic (6-fold) that statistically verification, although accomplished, was only done to satisfy the requirements of publication. It was obvious at this point that the pineal gland was a powerful endocrine organ at least in reference to reproductive physiology. The report of these findings appeared in *Science* in June 1965 (8) and it unequivocally

---

Received February 18, 1992.

"Remembrance" articles discuss people and events as remembered by the author. The opinion(s) expressed are solely those of the writer and do not reflect the view of the Journal or The Endocrine Society.

established the pivotal role of the pineal gland in photoperiodic alterations of reproductive function. Roger and I suspected, based on the work being concurrently conducted at NIH, that melatonin was the essential pineal signal in this response. At the conclusion of our paper we theorized the "pineal gland has the important function of regulating gonadal activity so that it is compatible with certain changing environmental conditions" thereby providing the foundation for the now well accepted fact that the pineal is essential in mediating fluctuations of reproductive capability in seasonal breeding mammals.

During these formative years, Hoffman and I visited Axelrod and Wurtman on a number of occasions to compare notes and commiserate about this remarkable gland. Physiologically, I and Ralph Hester (9) quickly showed that the interruption of the sympathetic innervation to the pineal gland destroyed its endocrine capabilities (the effects were equivalent to those of pinealectomy in terms of the reproductive system); we assumed that this was a consequence of the loss of the melatonin rhythm since it had just been shown that the sympathetically denervated pineal gland is no longer responsive to the LD environment (7). We additionally found that, unlike many other endocrine organs, the transplantation of the pineal gland to another site (in this case, under the renal capsule) rendered the gland endocrinologically inept even though the cells grew and appeared healthy (10).

Despite the remarkable associations between the pineal gland and the neuroendocrine-reproductive axis that we had uncovered, skepticism ran high in the scientific community relative to the physiological importance of the pineal gland. There was undoubtedly a variety of reasons for this, the major one of which was likely the fact that endocrinologists had been inculcated for decades with the idea that the pineal gland was functionless. However, there were other reasons as well. We had unfortunately made our observations using what was considered at the time to be an unusual species, that is, we had not used the albino rat. Many scientists questioned (I recall these discussions to this day) whether findings obtained in a pigmented, virtually tailless mammal with large cheek pouches could possibly contribute to our understanding of the endocrine system. Surprisingly, another bias surfaced that we did not suspect. Endocrinologists at the time were under the assumption that the pinealectomy procedure, which required opening the skull, was a severe surgical technique which certainly resulted in the near total maceration of the brain. Thus, they assumed any observed effect of pinealectomy would be meaningless and a nonspecific response to neural damage.

This came to a head when in 1966 I presented a paper at a scientific meeting in San Francisco where I described our experiences on the interactions of light and the pineal gland in controlling reproductive physiology in the hamster. I diligently went through the details and carefully described how pinealectomy prevented gonadal regression after the exposure of the animals to short days. Almost before I finished my presentation, a prominent scientist (who is still active and therefore will remain nameless) jumped to his feet and queried, is it not likely that the gonads of the short day exposed hamsters underwent atrophy because when they are pinealectomized much of the brain is destroyed and the neuroendocrine-reproductive axis therefore became nonfunctional? He clearly had let his bias enter into his interpretation of the data since pinealectomy had not induced gonadal regression but had, to the contrary, prevented it, that is, restored normal reproductive function. When I reminded him of this, he acted startled and quickly returned to his seat. Very early, Hoffman and I had perfected a pinealectomy method which protected the brain from damage when the gland is removed (11).

Not everyone was skeptical, however. Theodore Schwartz readily reviewed some of our early papers for the Yearbook of Endocrinology. Other noteworthy scientists quickly recognized the importance of the work and invited me to their respective institutions to "strut my stuff"; in particular, I recall Ernie Knobil (then at the University of Pittsburgh), Bill Hansel at Cornell, and Vernon Mountcastle at Johns Hopkins issued such invitations.

The 1960s were clearly exciting times for the pineal gland. Many of the basic biochemical and endocrine aspects of the gland were exposed during these formative years. The status of research on the pineal at the end of the decade can be found in two reviews that appeared at the time and which summarize both the biosynthetic properties and endocrine capabilities of this remarkable organ (12, 13). Since then, research on the pineal gland has progressed rapidly and it has attracted an increasingly larger number of scientists. It has indeed been established as a legitimate organ of internal secretion with an important position in the neuroendocrine hierarchy. I and my colleagues no longer have to take a defensive position when we mention the pineal gland and its ubiquitously acting hormone, melatonin.

Russel J. Reiter
Department of Cellular and Structural Biology
The University of Texas
Health Science Center at San Antonio

References

1. **Lerner AB, Case JD, Takahashi Y, Lee TH, Mori W** 1958 Isolation of melatonin, the pineal factor that lightens melanocytes. J Am Chem Soc 80:2587
2. **Lerner AB, Case JD, Heinzelman RV** 1959 Structure of melatonin. J Am Chem Soc 81:6084
3. **Axelrod J, Weissbach H** 1960 Enzymatic O-methylation of N-acetylserotonin to melatonin. Science 131:1312

4. **Axelrod J, Weissbach H** 1961 Purification and properties of hydroxyindole-O-methyltransferase. J Biol Chem 236:211–213
5. **Quay WB** 1963 Circadian rhythm in rat pineal serotonin and its modifications by estrous cycle and photoperiod. Gen Comp Endocrinol 3:473–479
6. **Wurtman RJ, Axelrod J, Phillips LS** 1963 Melatonin synthesis in the pineal gland: control by light. Science 142:1071–1073
7. **Axelrod J, Wurtman RJ, Snyder SH** 1965 Control of hydroxyindole-O-methyltransferase activity in the rat pineal gland by environmental lighting. J Biol Chem 240:949–954
8. **Hoffman RA, Reiter RJ** 1965 Pineal gland: influence on gonads of male hamsters. Science 148:1609–1611
9. **Reiter RJ, Hester RJ** 1966 Interrelationships of the pineal gland, the superior cervical ganglia and the photoperiod in the regulation of the endocrine systems of hamsters. Endocrinology 79:1168–1170
10. **Reiter RJ** 1967 The effect of pinealectomy, pineal grafts and denervation of the pineal gland on the reproductive organs of male hamsters. Neuroendocrinology 2:138–146
11. **Hoffman RA, Reiter RJ** 1965 Rapid pinealectomy in hamsters and other small rodents. Anat Rec 153:19–22
12. **Wurtman RJ, Axelrod J, Kelly DE** 1968 The Pineal. Academic Press, New York
13. **Reiter RJ, Fraschini F** 1969 Endocrine aspects of the mammalian pineal gland: a review. Neuroendocrinology 5:219–255

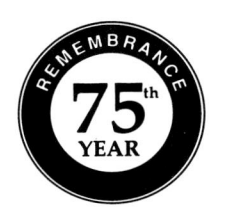

Remembrance: The Discovery of Growth Hormone (GH)-Releasing Hormone and GH Release-Inhibiting Hormone

In contrast to the other pituitary hormones, there was little information pertaining to a possible hypothalamic control of GH. In 1961, Reichlin (1) reported that basal hypothalamic lesions in rats interfered with growth and lowered the content of GH in the pituitary gland which suggested hypothalamic control. Before that time, in the mid 1950s, the argument continued to swirl as to whether or not vasopressin was a CRF, and whether there was an additional factor called CRF. At that time I was asked by Schering Corporation (Bloomfield, NJ) to serve as a consultant in the search for a GRF. I made four trips to their laboratories in 1958 and spent a half day each time discussing methods to discover such a factor. After that time, I heard no more about the matter for several years.

In the early 1960s we were purifying the various releasing factors. We had obtained evidence for a GRF in crude extracts of pituitary stalk-median eminence tissue by measuring the effect of systemic injection of these extracts on the GH content of the pituitary as estimated by the only bioassay available; i.e. the tibial epiphyseal cartilage assay in hypophysectomized rats (2).

By this time we had already shown that injections of GH depleted pituitary GH and had postulated a short-loop feedback of GH to suppress its own release (3). We concluded that this action was at least partly at the hypothalamic level because we could also deplete pituitary GH and reduce anterior pituitary weight of rats by implanting GH into the region of the median eminence (4).

By 1964 we had fractionated large batches of stalk-median eminence extracts from sheep using a long Sephadex G-25 column and assayed the fractions for releasing factors which included LHRF, FSH-releasing factor, PRL-inhibiting factor, CRF, vasopressin, and GRF. The first paper on the purification of GRF was presented at the plenary session of The Endocrine Society in June 1965 (5) in New York and published in *Endocrinology* in that year (6).

In early 1965, I received two peptides, stated to be almost pure, from Schering for testing for releasing factor activity. We screened both of these peptides and one of them released only GH. We were very excited about the results and proposed to Schering a joint publication on the purification of GRF; however, we never heard anything further about the matter. When we were writing up the results, we discovered a prior paper on GRF published in 1962 by Franz, Haselbach, and Leibert (7). They reported that a purified GRF obtained from Schering Corporation would enhance growth of rats and cause the release of GH into the medium of pituitaries incubated *in vitro*.

In 1964, Deuben and Meites (8) demonstrated that median eminence extracts released GH from hemipituitaries incubated *in vitro*, whereas cerebral cortex extracts were ineffective. The *in vitro* studies of Meites and colleagues (8) which showed that hypothalamic but not cerebral cortical extracts released various pituitary hormones convinced us to switch to an *in vitro* bioassay using hemipituitaries. The key was the use of preincubation to eliminate the large background hormone release during the initial incubation of the glands. Using the *in vitro* system, we confirmed the location of GRF in several sequential fractions from the Sephadex column. By this time (1967), we had moved from Philadelphia to Dallas and Krulich had come back to work on the problem. One Friday he came to me very excited stating that we had an inhibitor in fractions which emerged from the column shortly after GRF. I was extremely skeptical and thought that this might be a toxic contaminant in the tubes. He confirmed the activity and we then ran three additional Sephadex columns where we found the activity in the same location. This convinced us that the inhibitor was real and we submitted the first paper on GH-inhibiting factor (GIF) and also demonstrated its separation from GRF (9). We further purified GRF and GIF on carboxymethyl cellulose (6,10).

We went on to study the effect of these factors on the content as well as the release of GH from pituitaries incubated *in vitro* and the effect of coaddition of the GRF and GIF, showing that they could antagonize each other (11). We also demonstrated that the factors acted only on GH, and not on other pituitary hormones (12,13).

In the meantime, the existence of both of these factors was not widely accepted. Schally's group obtained highly purified GRF (14); however, Guillemin and collaborators reported (15) that they could find neither GRF nor GIF after purification of basic hypothalamic extracts by gel filtration on Sephadex G-25. Basic extracts were not generally used before, or since, to extract peptides of this type and may have been used in this instance because these fragments were collected by John Beck in Canada; he was primarily interested in extracting GH from the pituitary which does require basic conditions. It was my view that they might have pooled the fractions containing GRF and GIF, thereby extinguishing the activities of both factors.

At the Tucson meeting on Releasing Factors in 1969, the existence of both GRF and GIF was called to question. It was claimed that these were artifacts of the tibial epiphyseal cartilage assay (16). At that time, we had already sent media from fractions incubated with hemipituitaries *in vitro* to Peake in Daughaday's laboratory, who had confirmed the GRF activity of the fractions by RIA of GH (17). After this meeting we confirmed and purified both activities by RIA of the GH released from the incubated pituitaries (18).

To localize the activities in the hypothalamus, frozen sections were cut through the hypothalamus in three planes at right angles to each other, extracted, and bioassayed for the various releasing factors and inhibiting factors. By this means GRF was located in the region of the arcuate-ventromedial nucleus and GIF in the median eminence and also in the suprachiasmatic region (18). These localizations were subsequently shown to be correct; the observations antedated the definitive localizations by immunocytochemistry (19,20).

Guillemin's group was very fortunate to be able to isolate and determine the structure of GIF using extract from only 500,000 sheep hypothalami. This was made possible by the development by Brazeau *et al.* (21) of an assay which was excruciatingly sensitive to the inhibitor, namely the 4-day monolayer cultured pituitary cell assay.

Both Guillemin and I were members of an international committee to rename peptide hormones and the names liberin for stimulatory factors and sequestrin for inhibitors had been proposed. Therefore, it was not surprising that Guillemin renamed GIF, somatostatin (SRIF) (21). It has never been shown to produce growth stasis, as expected from the name, since it is a very labile molecule. Thus, somatostatin is a misnomer. Because of its marked inhibitory action at many sites throughout the body, we proposed an alternative name, panhibin (22). Finally, the recently developed, long acting, highly potent analog of the peptide can produce growth stasis.

The breakthrough in GRF research was provided by Frohman, who discovered an extra-hypothalamic tumor which secreted GRF. Unfortunately, he did not isolate and determine structure of the peptide. Thorner uncovered a similar tumor and sent it to Vale at the Salk Institute for fractionation. Since this tumor contained manyfold more GRF than the hypothalamus and lacked SRIF and with the advances in peptide chemistry in the intervening years, Rivier, Vale, and their co-workers (23) were able to determine the structure of the human pancreatic GRF in 1982. However, Guillemin was fortunate to secure a similar tumor in France which he brought back to his laboratory also at the Salk Institute. His group (24) determined the structure from this tumor, which was identical to that obtained by Rivier *et al.* (23) except for the addition of four amino acids at the C-terminal end of the molecule. That compound constitutes the bulk of the GRH found in the human hypothalamus, although there is a small amount of the 40 amino acid GRH as well. Finally, 12 yr after the discovery of the structure of SRIF, the structure of GRH had been revealed.

Samuel M. McCann
Department of Physiology
Neuropeptide Division
The University of Texas
Southwestern Medical Center

References

1. **Reichlein S** 1961 Growth hormone content of pituitaries from rats with hypothalamic lesions. Endocrinology 69:225–230
2. **Krulich L, Dhariwal APS, McCann SM** 1965 Growth hormone-releasing activity of crude ovine hypothalamic extracts. Proc Soc Exp Biol Med 120:180–184
3. **Krulich L, McCann SM** 1966 Influence of growth hormone (GH) on content of GH in the pituitaries of normal rats. Proc Soc Exp Biol Med 121:1114–1117
4. **Katz SH, Molitch M, McCann SM** 1969 The effect of hypothalamic implants of growth hormone (GH) on anterior pituitary weight and GH concentration. Endocrinology 85:725–734
5. **Krulich L, Dhariwal APS, McCann SM,** Hypothalamic control of growth hormone (GH) secretion. Program of the 47th Annual Meeting of the Endocrine Society, New York, 1965, p 21 (Abstract)
6. **Dhariwal APS, Krulich L, Katz S, McCann SM** 1965 Purification of growth hormone-releasing factor (GH-RF). Endocrinology 77:932–936
7. **Franz J, Haselbach CH, Libert O** 1962 Studies of the effect of hypothalamic extracts on somatotrophic pituitary function. Acta Endocrinol (Copenh) 41:336–350
8. **Deuben RR, Meites J** 1964 Stimulation of pituitary growth hormone release by a hypothalamic extract *in vitro*. Endocrinology 74:408–414
9. **Krulich L, Dhariwal APS, McCann SM** 1968 Stimulatory and inhibitory effects of purified hypothalamic extracts on growth hormone release from rat pituitary *in vitro*. Endocrinology 83:783–790
10. **Dhariwal APS, Krulich L, McCann SM** 1969 Purification of a growth hormone inhibiting factor (GIF) from sheep hypothalamus. Neuroendocrinology 4:282–288
11. **Krulich L, McCann SM** 1969 Effect of GRF and GIF on the release and concentration of GH in pituitaries incubated *in vitro*. Endocrinology 85:319–324
12. **Crighton DB, Schneider HPG, McCann SM** 1969 A study of the possible interaction of LRF with other hypothalamic releasing factors at the level of the pituitary gland. J Endocrinol 44:405–410
13. **McCann SM, Dhariwal APS, Porter JC** 1968 Regulation of the adenohypophysis. Ann Rev Physiol 30:589–640
14. **Ali AV, Arimura A, Wakabashyi I, Sawano S, Barrett JF, Bowers CY, Redding TW, Mittler JC, Saito A** 1970 The chemistry of hypothalmic growth hormone-releasing hormone (GRH). In: Meites J (ed) Hypophysiotropic Hormones of the Hypothalamus: Assay and Chemistry. Williams & Wilkins Company, Baltimore, pp 208–226

15. **Roger NW, Beck JC, Burgus R, Guillemin R** 1969 Variability of response in the bioassay for hypothalamic somatotropin-releasing factor based on rat pituitary growth hormone content. Endocrinology 84:1373–1383
16. **Daughaday WH, Peake GT, Machlin LJ** 1970 Assay of the growth hormone releasing factor. In: Meites J (ed) Hypophysiotropic Hormones of the Hypothalamus: Assay and Chemistry. Williams & Wilkins Company, Baltimore, pp 151–170
17. **McCann SM** 1970 In: Meites J (ed). Hypophysiotropic Hormones of the Hypothalamus: Assay and Chemistry. Williams & Wilkins Company, Baltimore. Discussion to Ref. 16, pp 163–165
18. **Krulich L, Illner P, Fawcett CP, Quijada M, McCann** 1972 Dual hypothalamic regulation of growth hormone secretion. In: Pecile A, Muller EE (eds) Growth and Growth Hormone. Excerpta Medica International Congress Series, no 244, pp 306–316
19. **Elde R, Hökfelt T** 1979 Localization of hypophysiotropic peptides and other biologically active peptides within the brain. Ann Rev Physiol 41:587–602
20. **Bloch B, Brazeau P, Ling N, Bohlen P, Esch F, Wehrenberg WB, Benoit R, Bloom F, Guillemin R** 1983 Immunohistochemical detection of growth hormone-releasing factor in brain. Nature 301:607–608
21. **Brazeau P, Vale W, Burgus R, Ling N, Butcher M, Rivier J, Guillemin R** 1973 Hypothalamic polypeptide that inhibits the secretion of immunoreactive pituitary growth hormone. Science 179:77–79
22. **McCann SM, Krulich L, Negro-Vilar A, Ojeda SR, Vijayan E** 1980 Regulation and function of panhibin (somatostatin). In: Costa E, Trabucchi M (eds) Neural Peptides and Neuronal Communication. Advances in Biochemical Psychopharmacology. Raven Press, New York, pp 131–143
23. **Rivier J, Spiess J, Thorner M, Vale W** 1982 Characterization of a growth hormone-releasing factor from a human pancreatic islet tumour. Nature 300:276–278
24. **Guillemin R, Brazeau P, Bohlen P, Esch F, Ling N, Wehrenberg WB** 1982 Growth hormones-releasing factor from a human pancreatic tumor that caused acromegaly. Science 218:585–587

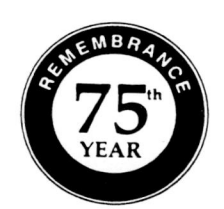

Remembrance for the Year 2016

With this brief note, the Remembrance series concludes. It began 18 months ago in order to provide a unique history of our journal and our society—and to celebrate the 75th anniversary of the journal. While thinking about the changes over 75 yr, it occurred to me that journal publishing will differ dramatically by the time the year 2016 (the 100th anniversary year of the journal) is with us. One can't paint a picture of what the journal might look like then—I have seen the "futuristic" car designs prepared in the 1920s—these are interesting only to the degree that one is amused by the embarrassment of the designer. It would be surprising, however, if the journal media itself (that is, the paper and ink) remain unchanged. This is a significant issue to us now, since each page we run over budget costs about $100. A few more magnetic bits might be cheaper.

In late 1987 and early 1988, with the help of a loyal group of Board members and an effective office staff, the time from submission to publication in *Endocrinology* dropped from nearly 12 months to 5.5 months. Almost immediately, the submission rate increased by 30% and by more than 60% over the next 2 yr. We expanded the pool of reviewers both on and off the North American continent—feeling that FAX and BITNET allowed all Society members to participate in the review process without slowing it down. Indeed, with more reviewers the decreased work burden was welcomed by many in North America. As the submission rate increased, so did the quality of submissions. Now came the first problem: with more submissions and a higher quality of same, shouldn't we be increasing the acceptance rate? Sure, but remember the $100/page overage cost? Clearly, we would have to use our pages more efficiently if we were to accommodate the reality arriving in the mail daily. We capped the number of references per article and down-sized the figures and type point sizes. These effected page savings of 2%, 6%, and 10%, respectively.

Midway into the effort, the Publications Committee allowed increased control by the Editors; we instituted editorials, and then, the Remembrance series. We added a color cover that changed monthly.

Now, as we prepare to enter 1993, the journal is robust with nearly 2000 submissions/yr and almost 7000 total published pages annually. Our board and reviewers in general (a group of 6000) are an international group reflecting the submissions (in 1991–1992, 47% of the submissions came from outside the U.S.) and the international makeup of our Society and discipline. The microscopic reflection of increased world-wide submissions was that we had to learn to accept bank card payments and bank transfers.

As those of you who read this in the year 2016 look back on our efforts, it is likely that they will appear modest compared to what you will be able to do—we did the best we could with just paper and ink! No matter how you are "publishing," we expect you will still hold the view that communication (journals and meetings) is what makes us a Society and a profession.

There is a story about a self-impressed individual whose autobiography was delayed when the typesetter ran out of the letter, "I." With this in mind, this editor has avoided inflicting himself upon you with any regularity. With this issue, however, the term of service of this office is completed and, for that reason, I want to take a moment to thank those who have been loyal reviewers, board members, office staff, members of the Publications Committee, those who have volunteered to be helpful, the redactory staff, and the editors. I offer my confidence that the new Editor-in-Chief and editors will expand the influence of the Journal.

P. Michael Conn

Received June 9, 1992.

"Remembrance" articles discuss people and events as remembered by the author. The opinion(s) expressed are solely those of the writer and do not reflect the view of the Journal or The Endocrine Society.